2,000 Toxicology Board Review Questions

2,000 Toxicology Board Review Questions

Richard J. Fruncillo, MD, PhD, DABT

To order additional copies of this book, contact:
Xlibris Corporation
1-888-795-4274
www.Xlibris.com
Orders@Xlibris.com
105054

CONTENTS

Chapter Name	Question Numbers	Page Numbers
1. Toxicologic Principles	1–54	11
2. Toxicologic Mechanisms	55–159	24
3. Absorption, Distribution, Excretion Of Xenobiotics	160–217	47
4. Xenobiotic Biotransformation	218–323	62
5. Toxicokinetic Theory	324–343	84
6. Carcinogenesis/Mutagenesis	344–420	91
7. Toxicology During Development	421–479	111
8. Immune System Toxicology	480–551	126
9. Hematologic Toxicology	552–611	143
10. Hepatic Toxicology	612–669	157
11. Renal Toxicology	670–716	171
12. Cardiovascular Toxicology	717–781	184
13. Dermal Toxicology	782–817	199
14. Neurotoxicology	818–883	209
15. Ocular Toxicology	884–912	224
16. Respiratory Toxicology	913–972	223

17.	Reproductive Toxicology	973–1,020	247
18.	Endocrine Toxicology	1,021–1,072	260
19.	Metal Toxicology	1,073–1,159	273
20.	Chemical And Solvent Toxicology	1,160–1,233	291
21.	Pesticides	1,234–1,312	308
22.	Animal Toxicology	1,313–1,366	325
23.	Toxicology Of Plants	1,367–1,451	336
24.	Radiation Toxicology	1,452–1,475	354
25.	Environmental Toxicology	1,476–1,511	362
26.	Air And Water Pollution	1,512–1,554	372
27.	Food Toxicology	1,555–1,615	383
28.	Occupational Toxicology	1,616–1,657	396
29.	Analytical Toxicology	1,658–1,690	405
30.	Drug Abuse Toxicology	1,691–1,790	414
31.	Medical Toxicology	1,791–1,917	440
32.	Epidemiology/Statistics /Risk Assessment	1,918–1,952	474
33.	Alcohol Toxicology	1,953–1,967	484
34.	Antidotes	1,968–1,984	490
35.	Toxicologic Disasters	1,985–2,000	494

DISCLAIMER

The clinical questions in this review book were chosen from some of the most recent and well-respected textbooks in the field. However, it is well-known that the standard of care in the practice of medicine can change rapidly. Every week, hundreds of clinically relevant new scientific journal articles are published worldwide. I am old enough to remember many examples of drugs that were indicated in the treatment of a certain disease at the beginning of my career that later became contraindicated. While I have made great efforts to ensure the accuracy of the information in this book at the time of publication, the possibility of human error still exists. Neither the author nor the publisher can guarantee that the information contained in this book is complete and accurate, and both disclaim any responsibility for any inaccuracies. Therefore, anyone using the clinical information contained in this book for direct patient care must absolutely confirm that it is still within the standard of care in their community. It is particularly important to check drug dosages, indications, interactions, and contraindications with the manufacturer's most recent product information. Also, the information in this book should not be interpreted by non-physician readers as "advice" for the treatment of drug overdose. Discussions with major poison-control centers are strongly recommended. Neither the author nor the publisher will assume liability for damages that result from the use of the information contained in any part of this book.

PREFACE

The purpose of this book is to learn toxicology. The information sources for these questions have come from many of the most recent authoritative textbooks in the area. I remember from my medical school days that the best way to comprehend the overwhelming amount of material presented was repetition in different formats. You needed to hear it in the classroom and on rounds, see it in texts, and as I found to be one of the most productive ways, review test questions. Till this day, I rarely forgot a piece of information that I answered incorrectly on a test and later looked up. Therefore, to receive the most benefit from this book, everyone is encouraged to read the reference text chapters, answer the questions in this book, and then reread the parts of the text referring to the test questions that were answered incorrectly. I have made every attempt to only have one *best* answer to each question. However, in a book of two thousand questions, there may be a few that are ambiguous. This book should be useful to those taking courses in general toxicology, to practitioners who would like a good recent review, and to those preparing for the various toxicology board examinations.

1

TOXICOLOGIC PRINCIPLES

1. A toxic substance produced by biological systems is specifically referred to as a _____.

    A. toxicant
    B. toxin
    C. xenobiotic
    D. poison

2. A newly formed hapten protein complex usually stimulates the formation of a significant amount of antibodies in _____.

    A. 1 to 2 minutes
    B. 1 to 2 hours
    C. 1 to 2 days
    D. 1 to 2 weeks

3. Prolonged muscle relaxation after succinylcholine is an example of a/an _____.

    A. IGE-mediated allergic reaction
    B. idiosyncratic reaction
    C. immune complex reaction
    D. reaction related to a genetic increase in the activity of a liver enzyme

4. Increased production of methemogloblin is due to a decreased activity of _____.

    A. cytochrome P450 2B6
    B. NADH cytochrome b5 reductase
    C. cytochrome oxidase
    D. cytochrome a3

5. The most common target organ of toxicity is the _____.

    A. heart
    B. lung
    C. CNS (brain and spinal cord)
    D. skin

6. The organs least involved in systemic toxicity are _____.

    A. brain and peripheral nerves
    B. muscle and bone
    C. liver and kidney
    D. hematopoietic system and lungs

7. If two organophosphate insecticides are absorbed into an organism, the result will be _____.

    A. additive effect
    B. synergy
    C. potentiation
    D. subtraction effect

8. If ethanol and carbon tetrachloride are chronically absorbed into an organism, the effect on the liver would be _____.

    A. additive effect
    B. synergy
    C. potentiation
    D. subtraction effect

9. If isopropyl alcohol and carbon tetrachloride are chronically absorbed into an organism, the effect on the liver would be _____.

A. additive effect
B. synergy
C. potentiation
D. subtraction effect

10. The treatment of strychnine induced convulsions by diazepam is an example of _____.

A. chemical antagonism
B. dispositional antagonism
C. receptor antagonism
D. functional antagonism

11. The use of antitoxin in the treatment of snakebites is an example of _____.

A. dispositional antagonism
B. chemical antagonism
C. receptor antagonism
D. functional antagonism

12. The use of charcoal to prevent the absorption of diazepam is an example of _____.

A. dispositional antagonism
B. chemical antagonism
C. receptor antagonism
D. functional antagonism

13. The use of tamoxifen in certain breast cancers is an example of _____.

A. dispositional antagonism
B. chemical antagonism

C. receptor antagonism

D. functional antagonism

14. Chemicals known to produce dispositional tolerances are
_____.

A. benzene and xylene

B. trichloroethylene and methylene chloride

C. paraquat and diaquat

D. carbon tetrachloride and cadmium

15. The most rapid exposure to a chemical would occur through
which of the following routes?

A. oral

B. subcutaneous

C. inhalation

D. intramuscular

16. A chemical that is toxic to the brain but which is detoxified in
the liver would be expected to be _____.

A. more toxic orally than intramuscularly

B. more toxic rectally than intravenously

C. more toxic via inhalation than orally

D. more toxic on the skin than intravenously

17. The LD50 is calculated from _____.

A. a quantal dose-response curve

B. a hormesis dose-response curve

C. a graded dose-response curve

D. a log-log dose-response curve

18. A U-shaped graded toxicity dose-response curve is seen in
humans with _____.

A. pesticides

B. sedatives

C. opiates
D. vitamins

19. The TD1/ED99 is called _____.

A. margin of safety
B. therapeutic index
C. potency ratio
D. efficacy ratio

20. All of the following are reasons for selective toxicity except _____.

A. transport differences between cells
B. biochemical differences between cells
C. cytology of male neurons versus female neurons
D. cytology of plant cells versus animal cells

21. Hereditary differences in a single gene that occur in more than 1% of the population are referred to as _____.

A. significant mutations
B. dominant mutations
C. genetic polymorphisms
D. sister chromatid exchanges

22. Which of the following statements is true?

A. Chemical carcinogens in animals are always carcinogens in humans.
B. A chemical that is carcinogenic in humans is usually carcinogenic in at least one animal species.
C. From a regulating perspective, carcinogens are considered to have a threshold dose-response curve.
D. Arsenic is an example of a chemical that is carcinogenic to humans and nearly all animal species treated.

23. The percentage of mating resulting in pregnancy is called
    _____.

    A. fertility index
    B. gestation index
    C. viability index
    D. survival index

24. The percentage of pregnancies resulting in live litters is _____.

    A. fertility index
    B. gestation index
    C. viability index
    D. survival index

25. The lactation index in rats is the _____.

    A. number of live births that breast-feed
    B. number of days an animal breast-feeds
    C. calories lost per day by a mother who breast-feeds
    D. percentage of animals alive at 4 days that survive the 21-day
       lactation period

26. Which of the following statements is false?

    A. There is good concordance between human and animal
       neurotoxicity assessment.
    B. The developing nervous system is insensitive to toxicant
       exposure.
    C. Monkeys can be used to test low-level effects of
       neurotoxicants.
    D. In vitro cell cultures can be used in neurotoxicity
       evaluation.

27. A severe cytokine response that progressed to systemic organ
    failure occurred in a phase 1 study involving the use of _____.

    A. an uncoupler of oxidative phosphorylation
    B. a COX-2 inhibitor

C. a CD 28 monoclonal antibody

D. a microtubule assembly inhibitor

28. It has been postulated that within the human genome, how much variability in DNA sequence exists between any 2 individuals?

A. 0.01 %

B. 0.1 %

C. 0.5 %

D. 1.0 %

29. Which of the following can be used to characterize a response to a toxicant?
A. proteomics
B. transcriptomics
C. metabonomics
D. all of the above

30. All of the following are true concerning animal carcinogenicity studies except _____.

A. Historic control data is never considered.
B. A rodent carcinogenicity study usually takes 2 years.
C. It is impractical to use doses that would occur in normal human exposure due to the large number of animals required.
D. Gender differences in background tumor incidence are sometimes observed.

31. Examples of significant concentrations of a toxicant in a tissue that is not a target organ include all of the following except _____.

A. lead in bone
B. DDT in adipose tissue
C. paraquat in lung
D. TCDD in adipose tissue

32. The ability of a chemical to cause acute skin and eye irritation is usually evaluated in a _____.

   A. rabbit
   B. rat
   C. mouse
   D. dog

33. Before a potential pharmaceutical compound can be given to humans, _____.

   A. an NDA must be filed with the FDA
   B. an IND must be filed with the FDA
   C. acute toxicity studies on 4 species must be conducted
   D. a 2-year dog carcinogenicity study must be completed

34. Phase 1 clinical trials are conducted to determine all of the following except _____.

   A. pharmacokinetics
   B. safety
   C. rare adverse effects
   D. preliminary efficacy

35. MTD stands for _____.

   A. minimal tolerated dose
   B. maximum total dose
   C. maximum tolerated dose
   D. minimum threshold dose

36. The acute toxicity study in animals provides _____.

   A. an approximate lethal dose
   B. information on target organs
   C. information on dose selection for longer-term studies
   D. all of the above

37. A subacute toxicity study in rats usually lasts _____.

    A. 3 days
    B. 14 days
    C. 3 months
    D. 6 months

38. The period of organogenesis in rats is _____.

    A. day 3 to 10
    B. day 7 to 17
    C. day 12 to 25
    D. day 17 to 56

39. A dose of investigational drug that suppresses body weight gain slightly in a 90-day animal study is defined by some regulatory agencies to be _____.

    A. LOAEL
    B. NOAEL
    C. MTD
    D. reference dose

40. A subchronic animal study required by the FDA will usually include _____.

    A. two species (usually one rodent and one nonrodent)
    B. both genders
    C. at least three doses (low, intermediate, and high)
    D. all of the above

41. When all receptors are occupied by a toxicant and there is a maximum amount of receptor-toxicant complexes, the response is labeled _____.

    A. t ½
    B. LCmax

C. Emax

D. Cmax

42. Which of the following statements is true?

A. Toxicant-receptor interactions are always reversible.
B. Receptors for toxicants are always enzymes.
C. The toxic response is related to the toxicant concentration in the plasma more so than the concentration at the site of action.
D. None of the above

43. An increase in free drug concentration will _____.

A. increase the pharmacologic effect
B. decrease the toxic effect
C. decrease the amount of drug filtered at the glomerulus
D. none of the above

Matching Test

44.	antagonism	A.	program to prevent birth defects
45.	TOCP	B.	performs human risk assessment
46.	probit unit	C.	idiosyncratic-prolonged apnea
47.	synergy	D.	delayed neurotoxicity
48.	succinylcholine	E.	normal equivalent deviation plus 5
49.	STEPS	F.	$4 + 0 = 1$
50.	Superfund Act	G.	toxicology and the law
51.	descriptive toxicologist	H.	$2 + 3 = 10$
52.	regulatory toxicologist	I.	performs toxicologic testing
53.	forensic toxicologist	J.	studies/treats human disease caused by toxins
54.	clinical toxicologist	K.	support to clean toxic-waste sites

CHAPTER 1 ANSWERS (REFERENCES)

1.	B (I)		37.	B (I)
2.	D (I)		38.	B (I)
3.	B (I)		39.	C (I)
4.	B (I)		40.	D (I)
5.	C (I)		41.	C (II)
6.	B (I)		42.	D (II)
7.	A (I)		43.	A (I)
8.	B (I)		44.	F (I)
9.	C (I)		45.	D (I)
10.	D (I)		46.	E (I)
11.	B (I)		47.	H (I)
12.	A (I)		48.	C (I)
13.	C (I)		49.	A (I)
14.	D (I)		50.	K (I)
15.	C (I)		51.	I (I)
16.	C (I)		52.	B (I)
17.	A (I)		53.	G (I)
18.	D (I)		54.	J (I)
19.	A (I)			
20.	C (I)			
21.	C (I)			
22.	B (I)			
23.	A (I)			
24.	B (I)			
25.	D (I)			
26.	B (I)			
27.	C (I)			
28.	B (I)			
29.	D (I)			
30.	A (I)			
31.	C (I)			
32.	A (I)			
33.	B (I)			
34.	C (I)			
35.	C (I)			
36.	D (I)			

REFERENCES

CHAPTER 1

I. D. L. Eaton and S. G. Gilbert, "Principles of Toxicology," in *Casarett & Doull's Toxicology: The Basic Science of Poisons*, 7th ed., ed. C. D. Klaassen (New York: McGraw-Hill, 2008), 11–44.

II. J. A. Timbrell, "Fundamentals of Toxicology and Dose-Response Relationships," in *Principles of Biochemical Toxicology*, 4th ed. (New York: Informa, 2009), 7–33.

2

TOXICOLOGIC MECHANISMS

55. A possible reason for the selective embryo/fetal toxicity of DES is _____.

    A. higher concentrations of free DES in embryo/fetus compared to adults
    B. binding to retinoic acid receptors
    C. lack of placental drug metabolism
    D. all of the above

56. The liver and kidney are major target organs of toxicity because _____.

    A. They both receive a high percentage of cardiac output.
    B. They both have substantial xenobiotic metabolizing capacity.
    C. They both have transport systems that can concentrate xenobiotics.
    D. all of the above

57. Acyl glucuronides are particularly toxic to the liver because _____.

    A. They selectively interact with macrophages releasing active oxygen.
    B. Active transport systems in the hepatocyte and bile duct system can greatly upconcentrate them.

C. They are resistant to glucuronidase.

D. They are suicide inhibitors of UGT2B7.

58. The selective renal toxicity of cephaloridine over cephalothin is due to _____ .

A. selective uptake by the organic cation transporter

B. selective inhibition of P-glycoprotein

C. selective uptake by the organic anion transporter

D. significantly less plasma protein binding of cephaloridine

59. All of the following are true of alpha-amanitin except _____ .

A. It is less orally available than phalloidin.

B. It inhibits RNA polymerase II.

C. It is transported into the hepatocye by a bile acid transporter.

D. It is a mushroom toxin.

60. All of the following are true of the toxic mechanism of paraquat except _____ .

A. Lungs accumulate paraquat in an energy-dependent manner.

B. Its entry into the lung is assumed to be via the polyamine transport system.

C. Similar molecules with smaller distances between nitrogen atoms do not enter lungs as readily.

D. Cytotoxicity to alveolar cells is caused primarily by interference with calcium channels.

61. Enzyme induction of phenobarbital is mediated through _____ .

A. aryl hydrocarbon receptor

B. PPAR alpha receptor

C. constitutively active receptor (CAR)

D. estrogen receptor

62. CAR is downregulated by _____.

    A. hypericum extracts
    B. acetaminophen
    C. aspirin
    D. proinflammatory cytokines

63. The pregnane X receptor _____.

    A. is a cytosolic receptor
    B. is involved in induction of cyp 3A4
    C. is primarily expressed in skin
    D. all of the above

64. Xenobiotic toxicity that occurs after repair and adaptive processes are overwhelmed include all of the following except _____.

    A. fibrosis
    B. apoptosis
    C. necrosis
    D. carcinogenesis

65. Amphipathic xenobiotics that can become trapped in lysosomes and cause phospholipidosis include all of the following except _____.

    A. ethylene glycol
    B. amiodarone
    C. amitriptyline
    D. fluoxetine

66. Which of the following parent toxicant-electophilic metabolite pairs is incorrect?

    A. halothane-phosgene
    B. bromobenzene–bromobenzene 3, 4 oxide
    C. benzene–muconic aldehyde
    D. allyl alcohol–acrolein

67. All of the following are capable of accepting electrons from reductases and forming radicals except _____.

A. paraquat
B. doxorubicin
C. n-hexane
D. nitrofurantoin

68. An example of the formation of an electrophilic toxicant from an inorganic chemical is _____.

A. CO to CO_2
B. AsO_4^{-3} to AsO_3^{-2}
C. NO to NO_2
D. hydroxide ion to water

69. The general mechanism for detoxication of electrophiles is _____.

A. conjugation with glucuronic acid
B. conjugation with acetyl CoA
C. conjugation with glutathione
D. conjugation with sulfate

70. The most common nucleophilic detoxication reaction that amines undergo is _____.

A. acetylation
B. sulfation
C. methylation
D. amino acid conjugation

71. Detoxication mechanisms may fail because _____.

A. Toxicants may overwhelm the detoxication process.
B. A reactive toxicant may inactivate a detoxicating enzyme.
C. Detoxication may produce a toxic by-product.
D. all of the above

72. The most potent carcinogen derived from nicotine is _____.

    A. naphthene
    B. styrene
    C. nicotine-derived nirtosamine ketone (NNK)
    D. meth tert-butyl ketone

73. Hydroxyl radical can be produced by all of the following except _____.

    A. the action of nitric oxide synthase on water
    B. interaction of ionizing radiation and water
    C. reductive homolytic fission of hydrogen peroxide
    D. interaction of silica with surface iron ions in lung tissue

74. If an electrophile is covalently bound to a protein that does not play a critical function, the result is considered a _____.

    A. toxication reaction
    B. detoxication reaction
    C. DNA adduct formation
    D. Fenton reaction

75. Which of the following receptor-exogenous ligand pairs is incorrect?

    A. estrogen receptor–zeralenone
    B. glucocorticoid receptor–dexamethasone
    C. aryl hydrocarbon receptor–rifampicin
    D. peroxisome proliferator activated receptor-clofibrate

76. Which of the following receptor-agonist pairs is incorrect?

    A. glutamate receptor–kainate
    B. glycine receptor–strychnine
    C. GABA (A) receptor–muscimol
    D. opioid receptor–meperidine

77. Which of the following receptor-antagonist pairs is incorrect?

   A. adrenergic beta 1 receptor–metoprolol
   B. serotonin (2) receptor–ketanserin
   C. glutamate receptor–ketamine
   D. GABA (A) receptor–avermectins

78. Clonidine overdose mimics poisoning with _____.

   A. morphine
   B. cocaine
   C. phencyclidine
   D. amphetamine

79. All of the following act as inhibitors of the citric acid cycle except _____.

   A. 4-pentenoic acid
   B. fluoroaceate
   C. DCVC
   D. malonate

80. All of the following are inhibitors of ADP phosphorylation except _____.

   A. oligomycin
   B. DDT
   C. ethanol
   D. N-ethylmaleimide

81. All of the following cause calcium influx into the cytoplasm except _____.

   A. capsaicin
   B. formate
   C. domoate
   D. amphotericin B

82. All of the following inhibit calcium export form the cytoplasm except _____.

    A. vanadate
    B. methylmercury
    C. bromobenzene
    D. carbon tetrachloride

83. Hydroxyl radical is enzymatically detoxified by _____.

    A. catalase
    B. glutathione peroxide
    C. glutathione reductase
    D. none of the above

84. Which of the following regarding cell death is true?

    A. Necrosis requires ATP.
    B. Release of cytochrome c usually triggers necrosis.
    C. Toxicants at low doses usually cause apoptosis and necrosis at higher doses.
    D. Apoptosis is never a desirable effect.

85. Blockade of voltage-gated potassium channels has been demonstrated with all of the following except _____.

    A. cisapride
    B. lorazepam
    C. terfenadine
    D. grepafloxacin

86. A drug that acts on potassium channels in pancreatic beta cells to impair insulin secretion is _____.

    A. terbutaline
    B. niacin
    C. diazoxide
    D. lidocaine

87. Chemicals cause major cell death by all of the following mechanisms except _____.

    A. rise in intracellular calcium
    B. ATP depletion
    C. inhibition of drug metabolizing enzymes
    D. overproduction of reactive oxygen species (ROS)

88. All of the following are inhibitors of cytochrome oxidase except _____.

    A. MPP+
    B. phosphine
    C. azide
    D. hydrogen sulfide

89. All of the following are inhibitors of NADH coenzyme Q reductase (complex 1) except _____.

    A. rotenone
    B. paraquat
    C. arsenite
    D. amytal

90. All of the following statements are true except _____.

    A. Macrophages can generate nitric oxide radical.
    B. Macrophages can discharge myeloperoxidase into phagocytic vacuoles.
    C. Nitric oxide radical is produced by the action of nitric oxide synthase on arginine.
    D. Superoxide anion radical and nitric oxide radical can combine to form the peroxynitrite anion.

91. A contributing factor in the termination of tissue regeneration is thought to be _____.

    A. depletion of local ATP
    B. plateau of protein synthesis regulated by DNA

C. accumulation of hypochlorous acid, which is a potent antimitrogen

D. dominance of TGF beta over mitogens

92. Overexpression of the divalent metal transporter 1 in iron deficiency will lead to increased intestinal absorption of _____.

A. cadmium and lead
B. sodium and calcium
C. potassium and magnesium
D. lithium and aluminum

93. An intracellular protein that increases ATP production and decreases ATP consumption is _____.

A. ras
B. BAX
C. AMPK
D. VEGF

94. The heat-shock response and endoplasmic reticulum stress response both _____.

A. repair damaged DNA
B. repair misfolded proteins
C. repair damaged lipids
D. all of the above

95. Free radicals can be produced in inflammed tissue by the action of all of the following enzymes except _____.

A. aconitase
B. NADPH oxidase
C. nitric oxide synthase
D. myeloperoxidase

96. All of the following are elements of the hypoxia response except
    _____.

    A. production of HIF-1alpha
    B. production of erythropoetin
    C. production of proteins that stimulate aerobic ATP synthesis
       from glucose
    D. production of growth factors that stimulate angiogenesis

97. An example of a protein that results from a mutation of an
    oncogene is _____.

    A. ICAM-I
    B. ras
    C. STAT
    D. C/EBP

98. All of the following are mitogenic growth factors except _____.

    A. HGF
    B. TGF alpha
    C. CTGF
    D. noxa

99. If only a few mitochondria are injured in a cell, the outcome
    _____.

    A. can be cell survival
    B. will always be both cellular apoptosis and necrosis
    C. will always be apoptosis
    D. will always be necrosis

100. Mechanisms opposing distribution of a toxicant to a target tissue
     include all of the following except _____.

    A. plasma protein binding
    B. blood-brain barrier
    C. distribution to nontarget organ storage site
    D. cellular uptake transporters on target tissues

101. Nonvolatile, highly lipid-soluble chemicals that are resistant to biotransformation are eliminated from the body by all of the following processes except _____.

    A. excretion in bile
    B. excretion in breast milk
    C. exhalation
    D. intestinal excretion

102. Examples of parent xenobiotics that act as ultimate toxicants include all of the following except _____.

    A. lead
    B. carbon tetrachloride
    C. tetrodotoxin
    D. carbon monoxide

103. Examples of xenobiotics whose metabolites act as ultimate toxicants include all of the following except _____.

    A. hexane
    B. TCDD
    C. ethylene glycol
    D. acetaminophen

104. Examples of noncovalent binding of toxicants to target tissues include all of the following except _____.

    A. binding of strychnine to glycine receptor
    B. binding of hydroxyl radicals to DNA bases
    C. binding of phorbol esters to protein kinase C
    D. binding of warfarin to vitamin K 2, 3-epoxide reductase

105. The reaction of hydrogen peroxide with a protein thiol group produces ____.

    A. carbon dioxide and water
    B. a protein sulfenic acid

C. a protein nitrosamine

D. cleavage of the peptide bond

106. Major target molecules for toxicants include all of the following except _____.

   A. proteins
   B. vitamins
   C. DNA
   D. lipids

107. All of the following toxins act by enzymatic action except _____.

   A. ricin
   B. anthrax
   C. tetrodotoxin
   D. botulinum

108. Apoptotic pathways can be initiated by _____.

   A. DNA damage
   B. mitochondrial insult
   C. death-receptor stimulation
   D. all of the above

109. The enzyme that repairs oxidized protein thiols is called _____.

   A. HMG-coenzyme A reductase
   B. adenyl cyclase
   C. phospholipase
   D. none of the above

110. The mechanism of action for bleomycin-induced lung injury is presumed to include _____.

   A. DNA-adduct formation
   B. generation of reactive oxygen species
   C. inhibition of cytochrome oxidase
   D. none of the above

111. All of the following are true of oxidative DNA damage except
_____.

   A. Mitochondrial DNA is much more resistant to damage than nuclear DNA.
   B. 8-hydroxy-deoxyguanosine in the urine is a marker.
   C. It can lead to base pair transversions.
   D. It can lead to a point mutation.

112. An example of a denatured protein is _____.

   A. Golgi complex
   B. micronuclei
   C. Heinz body
   D. histone

113. An important feature of lipid peroxidation is _____.

   A. It cannot be blocked by antioxidants.
   B. Damage can be propagated in a chain reaction-like manner.
   C. It never involves the Fenton reaction.
   D. The end products are different from the end products of the reaction of lipids with ozone.

114. All of the following are true regarding mechanisms of immune system toxicology except _____.

   A. TCDD-induced thymic atrophy may be mediated by the aryl hydrocarbon receptor.
   B. The addition of a hapten to a protein may cause a conformational change that displays previously hidden antigenic regions.
   C. Oral exposure of a xenobiotic is associated with a much greater chance of an immune reaction than by other routes.
   D. The "danger hypothesis" refers to a break in immune tolerance to an antigen triggered by signals initiated by cellular or systemic stress.

115. Which statement is true regarding the PPAR alpha-receptor?

    A. Stimulation causes peroxisome proliferation in humans.
    B. They are present in adipose tissue.
    C. They are involved in fatty acid beta-oxidation.
    D. Thiazolidinediones act as ligands.

116. Alterations in retinoic acid receptor (RAR) function have been associated with _____.

    A. cardiac and vascular toxicity
    B. CNS and peripheral nerve toxicity
    C. hepatic and renal toxicity
    D. embryo and testicular toxicity

117. Proteins present in brown adipose tissue act mechanistically like _____.

    A. pentachlorophenol
    B. rotenone
    C. cyanide
    D. doxorubicin

118. Which of the following regarding glutathione is false?

    A. It can act nonenzymatically as a radical scavenger.
    B. It is a dipeptide.
    C. Its levels can be upregulated in response to a need.
    D. It is a substrate for glutathione peroxidase.

119. All of the following are associated with necrosis except _____.

    A. requirement of ATP
    B. cell swelling
    C. association with an inflammatory response
    D. initiation by plasma membrane permeability changes

120. Another name for apoptosis is _____.

    A. passive cell death
    B. accidental cell death
    C. programmed cell death
    D. immune cell death

121. All of the following are true of apoptosis except _____.

    A. Cell membrane remains intact.
    B. Early in the process, capases are activated.
    C. Oxidative stress can initiate it.
    D. It can lead to carcinogenesis.

122. A mitochondrial factor involved in the process of apoptosis is _____.

    A. cytochrome a3
    B. cytochrome b6
    C. cytochrome c
    D. cytochrome a1

123. A class of drugs that can induce apoptosis in certain cancer cells is _____.

    A. barbiturates
    B. digitalis glycosides
    C. protein pump inhibitors
    D. COX-2 inhibitors

124. Which of the following signal-transduction pathways–effect pairs is correct?

    A. ras/ERK–suppression of apoptosis
    B. JNK-mediate apoptosis
    C. p38–production of inflammatory cytokines
    D. all of the above

125. A drug that works by disrupting mitosis is _____.

   A. paclitaxel
   B. doxorubicin
   C. methotrexate
   D. cyclophosphamide

126. Galacosamine causes _____.

   A. proximal tubular change
   B. focal liver necrosis
   C. peripheral neuropathy
   D. all of the above

127. Practolol was withdrawn from use because of _____.

   A. unpredictable beta blockade
   B. rebound hypertension
   C. teratogenicity
   D. oculomucutaneous syndrome

128. All of the following can inhibit opening of the mitochondrial permeability transition pore (mPT) except _____.

   A. cyclosporin A
   B. hydrophobic bile acids
   C. L-deprenyl
   D. bongkrekic acid

129. Microcystins target _____.

   A. adenyl cyclase
   B. phosphodiesterase
   C. protein phosphatase
   D. guanyl cyclase

130. All of the following are true of cytokines except _____.

    A. short half-life
    B. act locally
    C. produced in specialized organs
    D. have complex interactions

131. Molecular chaperones _____.

    A. repair denatured proteins
    B. repair damaged DNA
    C. repair damaged transfer RNA
    D. act as catalysts for new protein synthesis

132. Lipid repair ____.

    A. cannot occur
    B. requires NADPH
    C. may involve catalase
    D. none of the above

133. In peripheral neurons with damaged axons, repair _____.

    A. can only occur until approximately age 5
    B. follows the same mechanism as CNS repair
    C. requires activated neutrophils and astrocytes
    D. requires macrophages and Schwann cells

134. Apoptosis is most advantageous in ____.

    A. neoplastic prostate cells
    B. female germ cells
    C. cardiac myocytes
    D. CNS neurons

135. The principal factor leading to fibrogenesis is _____ .

    A. IL-8
    B. TNF alpha
    C. TGF beta
    D. IL-1

136. Fibrosis is harmful because _____ .

    A. It may compress blood vessels.
    B. It may contribute to tissue malnutrition.
    C. It may interfere with mechanical organ function.
    D. all of the above

137. All of the following are true regarding idiosyncratic drug reactions except _____ .

    A. They are rare.
    B. They are predictable from the pharmacology of the drug.
    C. The reaction can be dose independent.
    D. They involve genetic or acquired factors that increase susceptibility.

138. All of the following would indicate initiation of a cellular stress response except _____ .

    A. downregulation of DNA repair enzymes
    B. induction of apoptosis
    C. upregulation of antioxidant mechanisms
    D. stimulation of an immune response

139. All of the following contribute to organ-selective toxicity except ____ .

    A. organ-selective uptake
    B. tissue-specific expression of transcription factors
    C. number of chromosomes in nucleus
    D. tissue-specific receptors

140. The nephrotoxic effect of mercury on the kidney is thought to be mediated by _____.

    A. blocking the effect of ADH on the collecting duct
    B. interfering with ionic charges on the glomerulus
    C. a dicysteinyl-mercury complex mimicking endogenous cystine
    D. interfering with chloride transport in the loop of Henle

141. An example of a soft neutrophile is _____.

    A. sulfur in glutathione
    B. phosphate oxygen in nucleic acids
    C. mercuric ion
    D. carboxylate anion

142. The Fenton reaction produces _____.

    A. phosgene from chloroform
    B. formic acid from formaldehyde
    C. nitrogen dioxide from ozone and nitrogen
    D. hydroxyl radical and hydroxyl ions from hydrogen peroxide

Matching Test

143. muscimol

144. benzodiazepines

145. clonidine

146. baclofen

147. bicuculline

148. theophylline

149. nicotine

150. clozapine

151. tecadenoson

152. yohimbine

153. cocaine

154. alpha-bungarotoxin

155. botulinum toxin

156. bromocriptine

157. haloperidol

158. reserpine

159. ergonovine

A. serotonin agonist

B. prevents vesicle dopamine uptake

C. inhibits norepinephrine uptake

D. direct nicotine antagonist

E. direct dopamine agonist

F. direct serotonin antagonist/ glycine uptake inhibitor

G. direct GABA (A) agonist

H. indirect GABA (A) agonist

I. alpha-2 adrenoceptor agonist

J. dopamine antagonist

K. direct GABA (B) agonist

L. adenosine antagonist

M. direct adenosine agonist

N. alpha-2 adrenoceptor antagonist

O. direct GABA (A) antagonist

P. agonist at neuromuscular junction

Q. inhibits acetylcholine release

CHAPTER 2 ANSWERS (REFERENCES)

55. A (I)	91. D (IV)	127. D (XII)
56. D (I)	92. A (IV)	128. B (VIII)
57. B (II)	93. C (IV)	129. C (XIII)
58. C (I)	94. B (IV)	130. C (XIV)
59. A (II)	95. A (IV)	131. A (IV)
60. D (II)	96. C (IV)	132. B (IV)
61. C (III)	97. B (IV)	133. D (IV)
62. D (III)	98. D (IV)	134. A (IV)
63. B (III)	99. A (IV)	135. C (IV)
64. B (IV)	100. D (IV)	136. D (IV)
65. A (IV)	101. C (IV)	137. B (XV)
66. A (IV)	102. B (IV)	138. A (XV)
67. C (IV)	103. B (IV)	139. C (I)
68. B (IV)	104. B (IV)	140. C (I)
69. C (IV)	105. B (IV)	141. A (IV)
70. A (IV)	106. B (IV)	142. D (IV)
71. D (IV)	107. C (IV)	143. G (XVI)
72. C (IV)	108. D (IV)	144. H (XVI)
73. A (IV)	109. D (IV)	145. I (XVI)
74. B (IV)	110. B (V)	146. K (XVI)
75. C (IV)	111. A (V)	147. O (XVI)
76. B (IV)	112. C (V)	148. L (XVI)
77. D (IV)	113. B (V)	149. P (XVI)
78. A (IV)	114. C (VI)	150. F (XVI)
79. A (IV)	115. C (VII)	151. M (XVI)
80. C (IV)	116. D (VII)	152. N (XVI)
81. B (IV)	117. A (VIII)	153. C (XVI)
82. B (IV)	118. B (V)	154. D (XVI)
83. D (IV)	119. A (IX)	155. Q (XVI)
84. C (IV)	120. C (IX)	156. E (XVI)
85. B (IV)	121. D (IX)	157. J (XVI)
86. C (IV)	122. C (IX)	158. B (XVI)
87. C (IV)	123. D (IX)	159. A (XVI)
88. A (IV)	124. D (X)	
89. C (IV)	125. A (XI)	
90. B (IV)	126. B (XII)	

REFERENCES

CHAPTER 2

I.   U. A Boelsterli, "Organ-Selective Toxicity," in *Mechanistic Toxicology*, 2nd ed. (Boca Raton: Taylor & Francis Group, 2007), 23–38.

II. Ibid., "Cellular Transport and Selective Accumulation of Potentially Toxic Xenobiotics," in *Mechanistic Toxicology*, 2nd ed., ed. U. A. Boelsterli (Boca Raton: Taylor & Francis Group, 2007), 39–62.

III. Ibid., "Bioactivation of Xenobiotics to Reactive Metabolites," in *Mechanistic Toxicology*, 2nd ed., U. A Boelsterli (Boca Raton: Taylor & Francis Group, 2007), 63–116.

IV. Z. Gregus, "Mechanisms of Toxicity," in *Casarett & Doull's Toxicology: The Basic Science of Poisons*, 7th ed., ed. C. D. Klaassen (New York: McGraw-Hill, 2008), 45–106.

V.   U. A. Boelsterli, "Xenobiotic-Induced Oxidative Stress: Cell Injury, Signaling, and Gene Regulation," in *Mechanistic Toxicology*, 2nd ed. (Boca Raton: Taylor & Francis Group, 2007), 117–176.

VI. Ibid., "Immune Mechanisms," in *Mechanistic Toxicology*, 2nd ed. (Boca Raton: Taylor & Francis Group, 2007), 251–280.

VII. Ibid., "Nuclear Receptor-Mediated Toxicity," in *Mechanistic Toxicology*, 2nd ed. (Boca Raton: Taylor & Francis Group, 2007), 309–340.

VIII. Ibid., "Disruption of Mitochondrial Function and Mitochondria-Mediated Toxicity," in *Mechanistic Toxicology*, 2nd ed. (Boca Raton: Taylor & Francis Group, 2007), 357–384.

IX. Ibid., "Mechanisms of Necrotic and Apoptotic Cell Death", in *Mechanistic Toxicology*, 2nd ed. (Boca Raton: Taylor & Francis Group, 2007), 185-208.

X. Ibid., "Activation or Disruption of Cellular Signal Transduction by Xenobiotics," in *Mechanistic Toxicology*, 2nd ed. (Boca Raton: Taylor & Francis Group, 2007), 341–356.

XI. Ibid., "Impairment of Cell Proliferation and Tissue Repair," in *Mechanistic toxicology*, 2nd ed. (Boca Raton: Taylor & Francis Group, 2007), 209–220.

XII. J.A. Timbrell. "Biochemical Mechanisms of Toxicity: Specific Examples", in *Principles of Biochemical Toxicology*, 4th ed. (New York: Informa, 2009). 293-408.

XIII. U.A. Boelesterli, "Covalent Binding of Reactive Metabolites to Cellular Macromolecules," in *Mechanistic Toxicology*, 2nd ed. (Boca Raton: Taylor & Francis Group, 2007), 221–250.

XIV. Ibid., "Cytokine-Mediated Toxicity," in *Mechanistic Toxicology*, 2nd ed. (Boca Raton: Taylor & Francis Group, 2007), 281–288.

XV. Ibid., "Types of Toxic Reactions," in *Mechanistic Toxicology*, 2nd ed. (Boca Raton: Taylor & Francis Group, 2007), 15–22.

XVI. S. C. Curry et al., "Neurotransmitters and Neuromodulators," in *Goldfrank's Toxicologic Emergencies*, 9th ed., L. S. Nelson (New York: McGraw-Hil, 2011), 189-220.

3

ABSORPTION, DISTRIBUTION, EXCRETION OF XENOBIOTICS

160. Toxicants most likely to be reabsorbed after being filtered at the glomerulus are _____.

   A. organic anions
   B. organic cations
   C. neutral polar molecules
   D. highly lipid-soluble molecules

161. A high urinary pH would favor the excretion of _____.

   A. organic acids
   B. organic bases
   C. neutral organic compounds
   D. none of the above

162. Diuretics can enhance the renal elimination of compounds that _____.

   A. are of molecular weight greater than 70 kDa
   B. are ion trapped in the tubular lumen
   C. are highly lipid soluble
   D. are highly protein bound

163. The amount of a volatile liquid excreted by the lungs is _____.

   A. inversely proportional to its lipid-water partition coefficient
   B. directly proportional to its vapor pressure
   C. directly proportional to its molecular weight
   D. inversely proportional to cardiac output

164. Kernicterus results from _____.

   A. enzyme induction leading to decreased glucocorticoid levels
   B. excess ingestion of foods containing tyramine
   C. displacement of bilirubin from plasma proteins
   D. malabsorption of fat-soluble vitamins

165. All of the following could influence the gastrointestinal absorption of xenobiotics except _____.

   A. pH
   B. intestinal microflora
   C. presence of food
   D. time of day

166. The rate of diffusion of a xenobiotic across the GI tract is proportional to all of the following except _____.

   A. hepatic blood flow
   B. surface area
   C. permeability
   D. residence time

167. Which of the following is not absorbed in the colon?

   A. water
   B. sodium ion
   C. glucose
   D. hydrogen ion

168. Nanoparticles are considered to have diameters smaller than
_____.

    A. 100 μm
    B. 10 μm
    C. 1 μm
    D. 0.1 μm

169. All of the following are true of nanoparticles except _____.

    A. They are capable of exposing the lung to a large number of
       particles.
    B. They are capable of exposing the lung to a large particle
       surface area.
    C. Because of turbulance, very few reach the alveoli.
    D. They are the focus of recent toxicologic research.

170. All of the following are significantly stored in bone matrix
except _____.

    A. lead
    B. diquat
    C. strontium
    D. fluoride

171. All of the following can cross the placenta except _____.

    A. heparin
    B. rubella virus
    C. spirochetes
    D. IGG antibody

172. Methylmercury crosses the blood-brain barrier by combining
with cysteine and forming a molecule similar to _____.

    A. glycine
    B. glutamine
    C. taurine
    D. methionine

173. Which of the following statements is true?

    A. The blood-brain barrier of a 70-year-old is more permeable than that of a premature infant.

    B. Chemicals/drugs can be excreted into the urine by active secretion.

    C. The kidney lacks cytochrome P450 enzymes.

    D. All mammalian placentas have the same number of tissue layers.

174. All of the following are true of breast milk except _____.

    A. Acidic compounds may be more concentrated in milk than plasma.

    B. Toxicants can be passed from mother to offspring.

    C. Toxicants can be passed from cows to humans.

    D. DDT, PCBs, and PBBs can be found in human milk.

175. Active transport is characterized by all of the following except _____.

    A. movement against a concentration gradient

    B. energy requirement

    C. nonsaturability

    D. competitive inhibition

176. All of the following are true of facilitated diffusion except _____.

    A. does not require energy

    B. movement against a concentration gradient

    C. saturability

    D. involvement of a carrier

177. A transport process that removes particles from alveoli is _____.

    A. phagocytosis

    B. phospholipidosis

    C. mediated through BCRP

    D. mediated through MDR1/P-gp

178. P-gp, MRP2, and BCRP on enterocyte brush-border membranes function as _____.

    A. influx transporters
    B. bile acid binders
    C. metal transporters
    D. efflux transporters

179. Substrates for P-gp include all of the following except _____.

    A. cyclosporin
    B. paclitaxel
    C. ethanol
    D. colchicine

180. The transfer of toxicants by simple diffusion from areas of high concentration to areas of lower concentration is called _____.

    A. Dalton's law
    B. Priestley's law
    C. Fick's law
    D. Henderson's law

181. The fluid character of cell membranes is somewhat dependent on the amount of _____.

    A. saturated fatty acids
    B. transmembrane proteins
    C. ion channels
    D. unsaturated fatty acids

182. Aqueous pores are primarily involved in the transport of _____.

    A. small hydrophobic molecules
    B. large hydrophobic molecules
    C. small hydrophilic molecules
    D. large hydrophilic molecules

183. The agent with the largest octanel/water partition coefficient is
_____.

    A. paraquat
    B. ethylene glycol
    C. acetic acid
    D. TCDD

184. In renal glomeruli, pores allow molecules to pass through that
are smaller than _____.

    A. 60 kDa
    B. 30 kDa
    C. 15 kDa
    D. 5 kDa

185. Most of the vital nutrients essential for fetal development are
delivered by

    A. simple diffusion
    B. facilitated diffusion
    C. active transport
    D. ion trapping

186. Most toxicants cross the placenta by _____.

    A. simple diffusion
    B. facilitated diffusion
    C. active transport
    D. ion trapping

187. All of the following protect the fetus from toxicant exposure
except _____.

    A. tight endothelial cell junctions similar to the blood-brain
       barrier
    B. multiple tissue layers in the placenta
    C. biotransformation ability of the placenta
    D. presence of transporter systems in the placenta

188. All of the following statements are true of the P-gp, Mrp2, Mrp4, and BCRP transport systems that contribute to the blood-brain barrier except ____.

A. They are located on the luminal side of the capillary endothelial cell.
B. They can efflux uncharged molecules.
C. They do not require energy from ATP.
D. Some can efflux anionic or cationic molecules.

189. All of the following statements are true of the blood-brain barrier except ____.

A. It is not fully developed at birth.
B. It is remarkably constant throughout all areas of the brain.
C. Lipid-soluble chemicals will penetrate faster.
D. Ionized chemicals will penetrate slower.

190. Elemental mercury is poorly absorbed orally because of ____.

A. large particle size
B. efflux transporters
C. formation of insoluble complexes with phosphate
D. all of the above

191. The higher pH of the infant GI tract causes infants to be more susceptible to ____.

A. reflux disease
B. toxic megacolon
C. methemoglobinemia
D. GI erosions

192. Grapefruit juice affects ____.

A. activity of CYP3A4
B. function of P-gp
C. absorption of lovastatin
D. all of the above

193. Species differences in GI absorption are due to _____.

    A. anatomic factors
    B. gastrointestinal pH differences
    C. differences in GI microflora
    D. all of the above

194. All of the following are true of absorption of gases in the lung except _____.

    A. Lipid solubility is more important than in GI absorption.
    B. Degree of ionization is less important than in GI absorption.
    C. Diffusion through cell membranes is usually not rate limiting.
    D. Very water-soluble molecules can be removed in the nose before reaching the lungs.

195. The most characterized transplacental carcinogen is _____.

    A. warfarin
    B. phenytoin
    C. diethylstilbestrol
    D. vitamin A

196. Enzymes in the intestinal microflora may hydrolyze conjugates of organic compounds with _____.

    A. UDP-glucuronic acid
    B. sulfate
    C. both
    D. neither

197. The process of hydrolysis of an organic conjugate in the gut and reabsorption of the liberated parent compound is called _____.

    A. gastric bypass
    B. enterohepatic cycling
    C. first-pass effect
    D. well-stirred effect

198. The substance with the highest bile-to-plasma concentration ratio is _____.

    A. arsenic
    B. albumin
    C. iron
    D. gold

199. All of the following are transporters involved in biliary excretion except _____.

    A. P-gp
    B. Mrp2
    C. Bcrp
    D. ras

200. The organ that receives the smallest percentage of cardiac output is _____.

    A. liver
    B. lung
    C. kidney
    D. skin

201. A major route for the excretion of TCDD is _____.

    A. urinary excretion
    B. exhalation
    C. diffusion into fecal fat
    D. saliva

202. Xenobiotics can enter the gut by all of the following mechanisms except _____.

    A. secretion across the gut wall
    B. patent ductus arteriosis
    C. elimination in the saliva
    D. elimination in pancreatic juice

203. The two major plasma proteins that bind xenobiotics are _____.

   A. ferritin and transferrin
   B. ceruloplasmin and retinal-binding protein
   C. albumin and acid glycoprotein
   D. gamma globulin and fibrin

204. All of the following are true of the lung except _____.

   A. It is a major barrier to the absorption of chemicals into the blood.
   B. It has a large surface area and a thin membrane.
   C. It is a major site of inactivation of certain peptides and prostaglandins.
   D. It has less capacity to metabolize foreign compounds than the liver does.

205. All of the following contribute to the blood-brain barrier except _____.

   A. low protein concentration of brain interstatial fluid
   B. tight junctions between endothelial capillary cell
   C. significant endocytosis
   D. presence of efflux transporters

206. All of the following are true of the binding of xenobiotics to plasma protein except _____.

   A. The total (bound plus free) concentration is related to efficacy while only the free concentration is related to toxicity
   B. Only the free concentration is available to distribute to tissues.
   C. Binding to plasma proteins could be saturable.
   D. Displacement interactions from plasma proteins could lead to toxicity.

207. An example of an uncommon covalent binding of a drug to a plasma protein is demonstrated by the drug _____.

   A. thiopental
   B. captopril

C. warfarin
D. digoxin

208. All of the following statements are true of the ABC family of transporters except _____.

A. They all require ATP.
B. They can bind 1 or 2 substrates.
C. P-gp is an example.
D. They are found only in liver and kidney in humans.

209. Which one of the following statements is true?

A. PAH clearance is a good indication of glomerular filtration rate.
B. Organic anions and cations are transported by separate systems in the proximal convoluted tubule.
C. Insulin clearance is a good indication of renal blood flow.
D. Biliary excretion is favored for molecules of MW 300 or less.

210. Which of the following is most likely to require active transport processes for uptake into cells?

A. charged molecules
B. large hydrophobic molecules
C. small hydrophobic molecules
D. small highly lipid-soluble molecules

211. Which of the following has the highest octanol/water partition coefficient?

A. paraquat
B. DDT
C. aspirin
D. atropine

212. A weak acid with a pKa of 4 would be what percent unionized at pH 1?

    A. 10 %
    B. 50 %
    C. 99 %
    D. 99.9 %

213. Which of the following agents is rendered more toxic by bacteria in the GI tract?

    A. 2, 6-dinitrotoluene
    B. benzene
    C. snake venom
    D. aniline

214. Which one of the following statement is false?

    A. There are no aqueous pores in tight cellular junctions.
    B. Glucose transport into the CNS occurs by facilitated diffusion.
    C. It is estimated that 5 % of human genes are transporter related.
    D. Metabolic inhibitors slow the rate of facilitated diffusion.

215. Which one of the following is false regarding interactions in metal transporter systems?

    A. Thallium can be absorbed by the iron transporter.
    B. Lead can be absorbed by the calcium transporter.
    C. Fluoride can compete with the glucose transporter.
    D. Lithium can compete with the sodium transport system.

216. Particles can be removed from the alveoli by all of the following except _____.

    A. high fever
    B. lymphatics

C. phagocytosis

D. mucociliary elevator

217. Which one of the following statements is true with respect to absorption of a toxicant through the skin?

A. The skin is incapable of xenobiotic metabolism.
B. High solubility of toxicant in a vehicle will increase skin absorption.
C. All toxicants penetrate the stratum corneum by passive diffusion.
D. There is little variability of dermal absorption between rodents and primates.

CHAPTER 3 ANSWERS (REFERENCES)

160. D (I)	196. C (I)
161. A (I)	197 B (I)
162. B (I)	198. A (I)
163. B (I)	199. D (I)
164. C (I)	200. D (II)
165. D (I)	201. C (II)
166. A (I)	212. B (II)
167. C (I)	203. C (II)
168. D (I)	204. A (II)
169. C (I)	205. C (III)
170. B (I)	206. A (III)
171. A (I)	207. B (III)
172. D (I)	208. D (I)
173. B (I)	209. B (I)
174. A (I)	210. A (I)
175. C (I)	211. B (I)
176. B (I)	212. D (I)
177. A (I)	213. A (I)
178. D (I)	214. D (I)
179. C (I)	215. C (I)
180. C (I)	216. A (I)
181. D (I)	217. C (I)
182. C (I)	
183. D (I)	
184. A (I)	
185. C (I)	
186. A (I)	
187. A (I)	
188. C (I)	
189. B (I)	
190. A (I)	
191. C (I)	
192. D (I)	
193. D (I)	
194. A (I)	
195. C (I)	

REFERENCES

CHAPTER 3

I.   L. D. Lehman-McKeeman, "Absorbtion, Distribution, and Excretion of Toxicants," in *Casarett and Doull's Toxicology: The Basic Science of Poisons*, 7th ed., ed. C. D. Klaassen (New York: McGraw-Hill, 2008), 131–160

II.   A.G. Renwick. "Toxicokinetics," in *Principles and Methods of Toxicology*, 5th ed., ed. A. W. Hayes (Boca Raton: Taylor & Francis, 2008), 179–230.

III. J. A. Timbrell. "Factors Affecting Toxic Responses: Disposition," in *Principles of Biochemical Toxicology*, 4th ed., (New York: Informa, 2009), 35–74.

4

XENOBIOTIC BIOTRANSFORMATION

218. A probe drug for human CYP2C19 activity is _____.

    A. mephenytoin
    B. valproic acid
    C. carbamazepine
    D. warfarin

219. All of the following are true of CYP2D6 except _____.

    A. It converts codeine to morphine.
    B. It is polymorphic.
    C. It is induced by quinidine.
    D. Poor metabolizers have a lower risk of lung cancer.

220. Aryl hydrocarbon receptor agonists include all of the following except _____.

    A. TCDD
    B. benzopyrene
    C. 3-methylcholanthrene
    D. benzene

221. Enzyme induction in humans has been associated with _____.

    A. osteomalacia
    B. hepatocellular carcinoma

C. cirrhosis

D. psoriasis

222. In metabolism-dependent inhibition of cytochrome P450, _____.

A. The parent compound is a potent inhibitor.
B. The metabolite must be a product of P450 catalysis.
C. The metabolite is a potent inhibitor.
D. The inhibition is always irreversible.

223. A compound that induces CYP2D6 is _____.

A. rifampin
B. dexamethazone
C. ethanol
D. none of the above

224. All of the following are considered phase 1 biotransformation reactions except _____.

A. hydrolysis
B. conjugation
C. reduction
D. oxidation

225. All of the following statements are true except _____.

A. Forms of epoxide hydrolase can exist in both microsomes and cytosol.
B. Gemfibrozil is conjugated with glucuronic acid before it is oxidized by cytochrome P450.
C. CYP2D6 and CYP2C9 metabolize over half of the drugs in current use.
D. Biotransformation can take place in the gut.

226. UDP glucuronyltranferases conjugate all of the following endogenous molecules except _____.

A. thyroid hormone
B. bilirubin
C. steroid hormones
D. parathyroid hormone

227. If codeine were given to a patient who was a 2D6 ultrametabolizer, the most likely result would be _____.

A. inadequate analgesia
B. higher-than-normal levels of morphine at 2 hours postdose
C. higher-than-normal levels of codeine at 4 hours postdose
D. higher-than-normal levels of oxycodone at 4 hours postdose

228. A victim drug is _____.

A. a drug whose clearance is determined mostly by a single route of elimination
B. a drug that induces neutralizing antibodies
C. a drug that is unstable in plasma
D. a racemic drug mixture where one isomer inhibits the metabolism of the other isomer

229. Terfenadine and ketoconazole are examples of _____.

A. enzyme inducers
B. perpetrator and inhibitor
C. victim drug and perpetrator
D. drugs with limited biotransformation

230. All of the following are true except _____.

A. Hyperforin induces CYP3A4.
B. Broccoli inhibits 1A2.
C. Grapefruit juice inhibits intestinal CYP3A4.
D. Drugs that inhibit transporters can help anticancer agents.

231. Levels of UDPGA and PAPS are lowered by _____.

    A. Saint-John's-wort
    B. phenobarbital
    C. rifampin
    D. fasting

232. An example of a pair of enantiomers in which one inhibits CYP2D6 and the other has little inhibiting activity is _____.

    A. R and S methadone
    B. R and S warfarin
    C. R and S mephenytoin
    D. quinidine and quinine

233. Which of the following biotransformation enzyme–subcellular location pairs is correct?

    A. alkaline phosphatase–cell membrane
    B. carboxylesterase-blood
    C. sulfotransferase-cytosol
    D. all of the above

234. The least likely biotransformation reaction that aniline would undergo is _____.

    A. halogenation
    B. aromatic hydroxylation
    C. N-acetylation
    D. N-glucuronidation

235. The proteins KEAP1 and Nrf2 _____.

    A. suppress CYP expression in response to inflammation
    B. induce enzymes in response to oxidative stress
    C. promote DNA methylations
    D. none of the above

236. All of the following are true of glutathione except _____.

    A. Germ cells and ovum have high levels.
    B. Conjugation of dibromoethane results in a mutagenic metabolite.
    C. Conjugation of electrophiles is a major means of protecting DNA.
    D. Conjugation always occurs enzymatically.

237. Phenobarbital _____.

    A. causes liver tumors in humans and rodents
    B. causes liver tumors in rodents but not humans
    C. causes liver tumors in primates but not rodents
    D. causes liver tumors in rodents and nasal tumors in humans

238. All of the following are hydrolytic enzymes except _____.

    A. carboxylesterase
    B. alcohol dehydrogenase
    C. cholinesterase
    D. paraoxonase

239. All of the following are true of epoxide hydrolyases except _____.

    A. They add oxygen to a double bond and form a 3-member ring.
    B. They are important in detoxifying electrophiles.
    C. They play a role in converting benzo[a]pyrene to a carcinogen.
    D. Some forms are inducible.

240. Nitroreductase plays an important role in _____.

    A. nasal epithelium
    B. lung Clara cells
    C. white blood cells
    D. intestinal microflora

241. A drug that undergoes sulfoxide reduction is _____.

    A. haloperidol
    B. chloramphenicol
    C. thalidomide
    D. sulindac

242. Under low oxygen tensions, reduction reactions can be catalyzed by _____.

    A. cytochrome P450
    B. NADPH quinine oxidoreductase
    C. cytosolic aldehyde oxidase
    D. all of the above

243. Quinine oxidoreductases are thought to play a protective role in _____.

    A. liver toxicity of microcystin
    B. bone marrow toxicity of benzene
    C. renal toxicity of aminoglycosides
    D. neurotoxicity of n-hexane

244. All of the following are mechanisms for removing halogen atoms from aliphatic xenobiotics except _____.

    A. Grignard dehalogenation
    B. reductive dehalogenation
    C. oxidative dehalogenation
    D. double dehalogenation

245. Oxidation of ethanol to acetaldehyde takes place in _____.

    A. cytosol
    B. microsomes
    C. peroxisomes
    D. all of the above

246. Reductive dehalogenation of carbon tetrachloride produces
    _____.

    A. phosgene
    B. chloroform
    C. trichloromethyl radical
    D. hydrochloric acid

247. Acetaldehyde is converted to acetic acid by ALDH2 in _____.

    A. mitochondria
    B. cytosol
    C. microsomes
    D. all of the above

248. Aldehyde oxidase and xanthene oxidoreductase contain _____.

    A. zinc
    B. molybdenum
    C. selenium
    D. copper

249. The major metabolite of nicotine excreted into the urine is
    _____.

    A. nicotinamide
    B. nicotine glucuronide
    C. cotinine
    D. niacin

250. Patients with Parkinson's disease have elevated levels of which
    of the following enzymes in the substantia nigra region of the
    brain?

    A. COMT
    B. aldehyde oxidase
    C. CYP2E1
    D. MAO-B

251. All of the following are true of myloperoxidase (MPO) except _____.

A. It is present in neutrophils.
B. It can be induced by cyanide ion.
C. It forms reactive metabolites of drugs that cause agranulocytones.
D. It is polymorphic.

252. All of the following are true of prostaglandin H synthase (PHS) enzymes except _____.

A. They are known as COX-1 and COX-2.
B. They can convert xenobiotics to carcinogenic metabolites.
C. They can be inhibited by drugs.
D. They mainly cause toxicity in tissues that contain a high concentration of cytochrome P450.

253. The reactions catalyzed by flavin monooxygenases are most similar to those catalyzed by _____.

A. MAO-A
B. cytochrome P450
C. UDP-glucuronyltransferase
D. xanthine oxidase

254. The highest levels of cytochrome P450 are found in liver _____.

A. endoplasmic reticulum
B. cytosol
C. mitochondria
D. peroxisomes

255. All of the following are true of cytochrome P450 except _____.

A. It places one oxygen atom in a water molecule.
B. It does not interact directly with NADPH.

C. It can strongly bind carbon dioxide.

D. During catalytic activity, it directly binds substrate and oxygen.

256. All of the following are substrates for CYP450 epoxidation except _____.

A. coumarin
B. chlorobenzene
C. carbemazepine
D. chloroform

257. All of the following are substrates for CYP450 heteroatom oxygenation except _____.

A. toluene
B. NNK
C. omeprazole
D. lansoprazole

258. All of the following parent–toxic metabolite pairs are correct except _____.

A. diclofenac–acyl glucuronide
B. ethanol–acetic acid
C. halothane–trifluoroacetylchloride
D. acetaminophen–N-acetyl-p-benzoquinone imine

259. Which of the following reactions could be mediated by cytochrome P450?

A. hydration of an epoxide
B. breaking a hydrogen bond
C. cleavage of a peptide bond
D. dehydogenation

260. All of the following are substrates that are converted by glutathione transferase to more toxic molecules except _____.

    A. dichloromethane
    B. dibromoethane
    C. aflatoxin B1 8,9 epoxide
    D. hexachlorobutadiene

261. Human glutathione transferase enzymes are present in _____.

    A. cytosol
    B. microsomes
    C. mitochondria
    D. all of the above

262. GSTP polymorphisms in humans can influence _____.

    A. response to chemotherapy
    B. susceptibility to cancer-causing agents
    C. probability of developing asthma
    D. all of the above

263. Thiosulfate sulfurtransferase (rhodanese) is a major enzyme involved in the detoxification of _____.

    A. hydrogen peroxide
    B. hydrogen sulfide
    C. hydroxyl radical
    D. nitrous oxide

264. Thiosulfate sulfurtransferace polymorphisms may play a role in _____.

    A. cirrhosis and pulmonary function
    B. dementia and multiple sclerosis
    C. congestive heart failure and rhabdomyolysis
    D. ulcerative colitis and amyotrophic lateral sclerosis

265. All of the following are true of amino acid conjugates of xenobiotics except _____.

A. Glycine, glutamine, and taurine usually form an amide linkage.
B. Aromatic hydroxylamines can react with carboxylic acid groups of serine and proline.
C. They are eliminated primarily in the bile.
D. Acetyl CoA can be involved.

266. All of the following are true for glutathione transferaces except _____.

A. A steroselective conjugation will most likely occur non-enzymatically.
B. They are present within the hepatocyte at high concentrations.
C. They are a family of enzymes.
D. They are present in most tissue.

267. An example of a substrate for a glutathione displacement reaction is _____.

A. 1,2-dichloro-4-nitrobenzene
B. 1-chloro-2,4-dinitrobenzene
C. trinitroglycerine
D. all of the above

268. An example of a substrate for a glutathione addition reaction is _____.

A. hexane
B. 2-propanol
C. β-propiolactone
D. formic acid

269. Glutathione conjugates can end up in the urine as _____.

A. mercapturic acid
B. glucuronic acid

C. glutaric acids
D. all of the above

270. All of the following compounds can undergo O, N, or S methylation except _____.

A. acetone
B. nicotine
C. L-dopa
D. 6-mercaptopurine

271. An example of a transesterification reaction is _____.

A. methyldopa to 3-O-methyldopa
B. 4 hydroxyestradiol to O-methyl-4-hydroxyestradiol
C. cocaine to ethylcocaine
D. histamine to N-methylhistamine

272. All of the following statements are true regarding acetylation reaction except _____.

A. It increases the water solubility of almost all molecules.
B. It is a major route of biotransformation of aromatic amines.
C. It is a major route of biotransformation of hydrazines.
D. It requires the cofactor acetyl CoA.

273. N-acetyltransferases are located in the _____.

A. microsomes
B. cytosol
C. mitochondria
D. peroxisomes

274. Slow acetylators of NAT demonstrate all of the following except _____.

A. peripheral neuropathy from isoniazid
B. systematic lupus erythematosus from procainamide

C. peripheral neuropathy from dapsone

D. decreased hypotensive response from hydralazine

275. In contrast to glucuronidation, sulfonation is _____.

A. a low-affinity, low-capacity pathway

B. a low-affinity, high-capacity pathway

C. a high-affinity, high-capacity pathway

D. a high-affinity, low-capacity pathway

276. Induction of sulfotransference enzymes by rifampin may be clinically relevant for _____.

A. warfarin

B. digoxin

C. ethinyl estradiol

D. all of the above

277. All of the following statements regarding sulfonation reaction are true except _____.

A. They can make a molecule less lipid soluble

B. They always detoxify a molecule.

C. Some drugs must be metabolized to a sulfonate conjugate to have a pharmacologic effect.

D. Morphine-6-sulfate is more potent than morphine in the rat.

278. All of the following statements are true regarding methylation except _____.

A. The process generally decreases the water solubility of the parent.

B. The process can mask functional groups that can be metabolized by other conjugation enzymes.

C. Inorganic mercury and arsenic can be dimethylated.

D. High methyltransferace activity may lower levels of homocysteine.

279. All of the following are methyltransferase enzymes except
_____.

A. SAM
B. COMT
C. NNMT
D. HNMT

280. All of the following are true of glucuronide conjugates of xenobiotics except _____.

A. They can be excreted in the urine.
B. They are formed from activated xenobiotics.
C. They are substrates for beta-glucuronidase in the intestinal microflora.
D. They can be excreted into bile.

281. All of the following are true of sulfonation reactions except _____.

A. They involve the transfer of sulfate.
B. They are catalyzed by sulfotransferaces.
C. The cofactor for the reaction is PAPS.
D. They are excreted mainly in the urine.

282. The number of UGT mammalian enzymes that have been identified is approximately _____.

A. 5
B. 12
C. 22
D. 58

283. Immune hepatitis from NSAIDs may be explained by _____.

A. binding of an acyl glucuronide to a protein forming a neoantigen
B. methylation of DNA and subsequent immune stimulation

C. cholestasis caused by the sulfonated parent

D. genetic sensitivity to a portion of the parent molecule

284. In addition to the cytoplasm, sulfotransferaces are present in mammals in the _____.

A. endoplasmic reticulum

B. mitochondria

C. plasma membrane

D. Golgi apparatus

285. All of the following statements are true except _____.

A. CYP3A4 is induced by CAR and PXR agonists.

B. AhR is expressed only in human liver and small intenstine.

C. Highly chlorinated chemicals are resistant to metabolism.

D. AhR partners with ARNT to induce CYP1A1 and CYP1A2.

286. Most conjugation reactions occur in the _____.

A. mitochondria

B. peroxisome

C. cytosol

D. cell membrane

287. An example of a metabolite of conjugation that is more potent than the parent is _____.

A. oxazepam glucuronide

B. propofol glucuronide

C. morphine-6-glucuronide

D. thyroxine glucuronide

288. All of the following are true of UGT enzymes except _____.

A. They are inducible.

B. They can use UDP-glucose as a substrate.

C. They are present in many tissues.
D. They are more subject to inhibiting drug-drug interactions than CYP450 enzymes.

289. All of the following statements are true except _____.

A. Acyl glucuronides of NSAIDs can be toxic.
B. Glucuronide metabolites of aromatic amines can decompose in acid urine to produce tumorigenic chemicals.
C. Crigler-Najjar syndrome is due to a defect in bilirubin conjugation.
D. Gilberts disease is due to increased glucuronidation of endogenous substrates.

290. Which of the following statements is true of CYP3A4?

A. It is affected more by genetic polymorphisms than environmental factors.
B. It can bind 2 substrates at once.
C. It is induced by ethyl alcohol.
D. None of the above

291. A human probe for activity of CYP2E1 is _____.

A. dextromethorphan
B. erythromycin
C. chlorzoxazone
D. midazolam

292. Cytochrome 2E1 _____.

A. requires cytochrome b5
B. is inhibited by cimetidine
C. is induced by 3-methylcholanthrene
D. all of the above

293. Substrates for human CYP2E1 include all of the following except _____.

    A. styrene
    B. chloroform
    C. aflatoxin B1
    D. vinyl chloride

294. Substrates for human CYP3A4 include all of the following except _____.

    A. lovastatin
    B. sirolimus
    C. halothane
    D. midazolam

295. Inhibitors for CYP3A4 include all of the following except _____.

    A. erythromycin
    B. mibefradil
    C. ketoconazole
    D. phenytoin

296. A compound that inhibits CYP2D6 is _____.

    A. rifampin
    B. dexamethasone
    C. ethanol
    D. quinidine

297. What type of reaction would be expected to be catalyzed by flavin monooxygenase?

    A. N-dealkylation
    B. S-oxygenation
    C. O-demethylation
    D. S-dealkalation

298. All of the following are substrates for CYP450-mediated heteroatom dealkalation except _____.

    A. caffeine
    B. styrene
    C. diazepam
    D. dextromethorphan

299. An example of oxidative desulfuration is

    A. parathion to paraoxon
    B. imipramine to desipramine
    C. codeine to morphine
    D. enalapril to enalaprilat

300. An example of oxidative deamination is _____.

    A. nitrobenzene to aniline
    B. DDT to DDE
    C. benzene to hydroquinone
    D. amphetamine to phenylacetone

301. An example of a reaction catalyzed by aldehyde oxidase is _____.

    A. N-hexane to neurotoxic metabolite
    B. butylated hydroxytoluene to butylated hydroxyanisole
    C. vanillin to vanillic acid
    D. aflatoxin B1 to toxic metabolite

302. Activity of cytochrome P450 can be surpressed by all of the following except _____.

    A. vaccination
    B. hypertension
    C. infection
    D. inflammation

303. Cytochrome P450 activity can be affected by _____.

    A. foods
    B. social habits (smoking, alcohol)
    C. thyroid disease
    D. all of the above

304. Cytochrome P450–mediated reactions include all of the following except _____.

    A. ester cleavage
    B. methylation
    C. dehydrogenation
    D. oxidative group transfer

305. CYP3A7 is present mostly in _____.

    A. adult human liver
    B. fetal human liver
    C. rodent liver
    D. human lymphoma cells

306. The CYP450 present in the lowest amounts in human liver is _____.

    A. CYP 2C9
    B. CYP 2D6
    C. CYP 3A4
    D. CYP 1B1

307. Which of the following CYP450 enzymes metabolizes many therapeutic drugs and is present in human liver and small intestine?

    A. CYP 2D6
    B. CYP 2C9
    C. CYP 3A4
    D. CYP 1B1

Matching Test

308. theophylline   A. substrate for CYP2A6

309. omeprazole   B. inducer of CYP2E1

310. aniline   C. inducer of CYP2D6

311. debrisoquin   D. inhibitor of CYP 3A4

312. alprazolam   E. inducer of CYP 1A2

313. diclofenac   F. substrate for CYP 1A2

314. bupropion   G. inhibitor of CYP 2C8

315. fluvoxamine   H. substrate for CYP 2E1

316. paroxetine   I. substrate for CYP 2C19

317. nicotine   J. substrate for CYP 2C9

318. beta-naphthoflavone   K. substrate for CYP 2D6

319. isoniazid   L. inducer of CYP 3A4

320. no known agent   M. inhibitor of CYP2D6

321. carbemazepine   N. inhibitor of CYP 1A2

322. mibefradil   O. substrate for CYP 2B6

323. gemfibrozil glucuronide   P. substrate for CYP 3A4

CHAPTER 4 ANSWERS (REFERENCES)

218. A (I)	254. A (I)	290. B (I)
219. C (I)	255. C (I)	291. C (I)
220. D (I)	256. D (I)	292. A (I)
221. A (I)	257. A (I)	293. C (I)
222. C (I)	258. B (I)	294. C (I)
223. D (I)	259. D (I)	295. D (I)
224. B (I)	260. C (I)	296. D (I)
225. C (I)	261. D (I)	297. B (I)
226. D (I)	262. D (I)	298. B (I)
227. B (I)	263. B (I)	299. A (I)
228. A (I)	264. D (I)	300. D (I)
229. C (I)	265. C (I)	301. C (I)
230. B (I)	266. A (I)	302. B (I)
231. D (I)	267. D (I)	303. D (I)
232. D (I)	268. C (I)	304. B (I)
233. D (I)	269. A (I)	305. B (I)
234. A (I)	270. A (I)	306. D (I)
235. B (I)	271. C (I)	307. C (I)
236. D (I)	272. A (I)	308. F (I)
237. B (I)	273. B (I)	309. I (I)
238. B (I)	274. D (I)	310. H (I)
239. A (I)	275. D (I)	311. K (I)
240. D (I)	276. C (I)	312. P (I)
241. D (I)	277. B (I)	313. J (I)
242. D (I)	278. D (I)	314. O (I)
243. B (I)	279. A (I)	315. N (I)
244. A (I)	280. B (I)	316. M (I)
245. D (I)	281. A (I)	317. A (I)
246. C (I)	282. C (I)	318. E (I)
247. A (I)	283. A (I)	319. B (I)
248. B (I)	284. D (I)	320. C (I)
249. C (I)	285. B (I)	321. L (I)
250. D (I)	286. C (I)	322. D (I)
251. B (I)	287. C (I)	323. G (I)
252. D (I)	288. D (I)	
253. B (I)	289. D (I)	

REFERENCE

CHAPTER 4

I. A. Parkinson and B. W. Ogilvie, "Biotransformation of Xenobiotics," in *Casarett and Doull's Toxicology: The Basic Science of Poisons*, 7th ed., ed. C. D. Klaassen (New York: McGraw-Hill, 2008), 161–305.

5

TOXICOKINETIC THEORY

324. Systemic availability of an orally administered toxicant is dependent on _____.

    A. gastrointestinal absorption
    B. intestinal mucosa metabolism
    C. first-pass liver metabolism
    D. all of the above

325. Which of the following statements is true?

    A. Renal clearance is equal to urine formation rate.
    B. Hepatic clearance cannot exceed hepatic blood flow.
    C. A process that increases free drug concentration will decrease hepatic clearance and increase renal clearance.
    D. Total body clearance equals dose divided by half-life.

326. A classic example of a drug inducing its own metabolism is _____.

    A. warfarin
    B. lovastatin
    C. carbamazepine
    D. theophylline

327. An example of a thermodynamic parameter used in physiologic, toxicokinetic models is _____.

    A. tissue partition coefficient
    B. alveolar ventilation rate
    C. cardiac output
    D. liver volume

328. Fick's law of diffusion _____.

    A. is a zero-order process
    B. is a first-order process
    C. applies to active transport
    D. requires energy

329. The method of predicting the toxicokinetic behavior of chemicals and drugs across species is called _____.

    A. Monte Carlo simulation
    B. benchmark kinetics
    C. allometric scaling
    D. linear regression kinetics

330. Which of the following is not theoretically possible?

    A. volume of distribution greater than volume of human body
    B. volume of distribution equal to blood volume
    C. total clearance equal to renal clearance
    D. bioavailability (F) greater than 1

331. A compartment in which uptake of xenobiotic is dependent on membrane permeability and total membrane area is called _____.

    A. perfusion limited
    B. diffusion limited
    C. blood flow limited
    D. ventilation limited

332. The alpha phase of an intravenously administered drug classically represents the _____.

    A. absorption phase
    B. elimination phase
    C. dissolution phase
    D. distribution phase

333. An advantage of a physiologic, toxicokinetic model over a classic model is _____.

    A. It may be able to predict tissue concentrations.
    B. It only has 2 compartments.
    C. The mathematics are less complicated.
    D. It can give a better estimation of bioavailability.

334. The hepatic clearance of a drug with a high hepatic extraction ratio is largely dependent on _____.

    A. drug protein binding
    B. hepatic blood flow
    C. drug-metabolizing enzyme activity
    D. intestinal blood flow

335. All of the following are true of saturation kinetics with increasing dose except _____.

    A. Clearance must decrease.
    B. Half-life can increase or decrease.
    C. Volume of distribution will decrease if there is saturation of serum protein binding.
    D. Volume of distribution will decrease if there is saturation of tissue binding.

336. All of the following are true of nonlinear kinetics except _____.

    A. Ratio of metabolites will remain constant with change in dose.
    B. Clearance will change with change in dose.

C. AUC will not be dose proportional.

D. Decline of xenobiotic is nonexponential.

337. All of the following are true of first-order kinetics except _____.

A. Steady state concentration is proportional to rate of intake.

B. Rate of intake will not change time to steady state.

C. Half-life is inversely proportional to clearance.

D. A change in half-life will not change time to steady state.

338. All of the following are true of first-order kinetics except _____.

A. The elimination rate constant increases with increasing dose.

B. A semilogarithmic plot of plasma concentration versus time yields a single straight line.

C. The concentration of xenobiotic in plasma decreases by a constant fraction per unit time.

D. The volume of distribution is independent of dose.

339. After _____, 93.8 % of a dose of drug is eliminated.

A. 3 half-lives

B. 4 half-lives

C. 5 half-lives

D. 6 half-lives

340. All of the following are components of the central compartment except _____.

A. liver

B. lungs

C. bone

D. kidney

341. Which of the following has the largest value of distribution?

A. chloroquine

B. ethyl alcohol

C. albumin

D. ethylene glycol

342. The common units used to express total clearance of a toxicant are _____.

A. mg/mL

B. mg/min

C. mL/min

D. mg/min·mL

343. In first-order kinetics, _____.

A. A constant amount of toxicant is removed per unit time.

B. AUC is not proportional to dose.

C. Half-life changes with increasing dose.

D. Clearance, volume of distribution, and half-life do not change with dose.

CHAPTER 5 ANSWERS (REFERENCES)

324. D (I)
325. B (I)
326. C (I)
327. A (I)
328. B (I)
329. C (I)
330. D (I)
331. B (I)
332. D (I)
333. A (I)
334. B (I)
335. C (I)
336. A (I)
337. D (I)
338. A (I)
339. B (I)
340. C (I)
341. A (I)
342. C (I)
343. D (I)

REFERENCES

CHAPTER 5

I.   D. D. Shen, "Toxicokinetics," in *Casarett and Doull's Toxicology: The Basic Science of Poisons*, 7th ed., ed. C. D. Klaassen (New York: McGraw-Hill, 2008), 305–326.

6

CARCINOGENESIS/MUTAGENESIS

344. Which of the following benign-malignant neoplasm pairs is incorrect?

   A. lipoma-liposarcoma
   B. hemangioma-angiosarcoma
   C. squamous cell papilloma–squamous cell sarcoma
   D. bronchial adenoma–bronchogenic carcinoma

345. All of the following are true of nongenotoxic carcinogens except _____.

   A. There is a threshold.
   B. They are mutagenic.
   C. They cause no direct DNA damage.
   D. They can be tissue specific.

346. All of the following are possible outcomes for initiated cells in the neoplastic process except _____.

   A. cell death via apoptosis
   B. immediate distant metastatic spread
   C. can remain in static, nondividing state
   D. can undergo cell division to increase population of initiated cells

347. The progression state of carcinogenesis _____.

A. is reversible
B. involves conversion from preneoplasia to neoplasia
C. does not involve DNA modification
D. always forms a carcinoma

348. All of the following are true of the promotion stage of carcinogenesis except _____.

A. multiple cell divisions are necessary
B. only a single treatment is needed
C. DNA is not directly modified
D. decrease in apoptosis may be a mechanism

349. The carcinogenicity of inorganic arsenic is unusual in that _____.

A. It causes cancer in humans, but probably not animals.
B. It causes different cancers in humans and animals.
C. It causes cancer in animals, but not humans.
D. It causes cancer in plants, but not animals.

350. The most prevalent oxidative DNA adduct is _____.

A. 5-hydroxyuracil
B. thymine glycol
C. 8-hydroxyguanine
D. 9-oxoguanine

351. Malignant neoplasms of epithelial origin are called _____.

A. sarcomas
B. fibromas
C. carcinomas
D. papilloma

352. Malignant neoplasms of mesenchymal origins are called _____.

   A. sarcomas
   B. fibromas
   C. carcinomas
   D. papilloma

353. A carcinogen is an agent that when administered to animals _____.

   A. increases the incidence of malignant neoplasms
   B. increased the incidence of benign neoplasms
   C. increases the incidence of background neoplasms
   D. all of the above

354. An IARC carcinogenic classification of 2A means _____.

   A. The chemical is probably carcinogenic in humans.
   B. Animal data is positive for cancer development.
   C. Human epidemiology data is suggestive of cancer causation.
   D. all of the above

355. Which of the following occupational carcinogen–cancer type pairs is incorrect?

   A. formaldehyde-astrocytoma
   B. arsenic–skin cancer
   C. nickel–nasal sinus cancer
   D. benzidine–bladder carcinoma

356. The development of tumors in rodents after the implantation of solid materials is known as _____.

   A. multiple-hit carcinogenesis
   B. solid-state carcinogenesis
   C. single-hit carcinogenesis
   D. nonmutational carcinogenesis

357. Alpha 2μ globulin nephropathy from hydrocarbons and gastric neuroendocrine cell neoplasia from omeprazole are examples of neoplastic effects in rodents with _____.

A. no significance to humans
B. some evidence for human cancer association
C. strong evidence for human cancer association
D. IARC 2B classification in humans

358. Cosmetic preparations applied to the skin of the SKH1 albino hairless mouse would likely involve a test for _____.

A. tumor progression
B. solid-state carcinogenesis
C. photochemical carcinogenesis
D. anticarcinogenesis

359. The Syrian hamster embryo (SHE) assay is an example of a/an _____.

A. in vivo assay
B. 2-year bioaassay
C. organ-specific assay
D. transformation assay

360. In a classic experimental demonstration of cancer development in mouse skin, croton oil was used as _____.

A. an initiator
B. a promoter
C. a vehicle
D. a placebo

361. All of the following are true of the chronic (2-year) carcinogenicity bioassay except _____.

A. FDA mandates use of dogs and monkeys.
B. A vehicle control and 2 or 3 doses of test chemical are used.

    C. Male and female animals are used.

    D. At necropsy, the number, location, and pathology of each tumor are assessed.

362. Which of the following lifestyle-cancer associations is incorrect?

    A. dietary fat–melanoma
    B. tobacco smoking–bladder cancer
    C. ethanol–oral cancer
    D. moldy food–liver cancer

363. Which of the following drug-cancer associations is incorrect?

    A. thorotrast–angiosarcoma of the liver
    B. phenacetin–carcinoma of renal pelvis
    C. diethylstilbestrol–clear cell vaginal carcinoma
    D. estrogens–prostate cancer

364. Which of the following tumor suppressor gene–neoplasm pairs is incorrect?

    A. p16-melanoma
    B. Rb1–small cell lung carcinoma
    C. BRCA1-osteosarcoma
    D. WT-1–lung cancer

365. All of the following are true of the p53 gene except _____.

    A. It is essential for checkpoint control during cell division.
    B. The active form is a hexamer of 6 identical units.
    C. Enhanced MDM2 in tumor cells decreases functional p53.
    D. Mutations are associated with lung, colon, and breast cancer.

366. All of the following are true of carcinogens that initially at lower doses demonstrate protection against carcinogenesis except _____.

    A. induction of P450 enzymes as a possible mechanism
    B. exhibit a J-shaped dose-response curve

   C. stimulation of adaptive responses that dominate at low doses

   D. a mechanism that is only exhibited by tumor promoters

367. Which of the following chemoprotective agent–mechanism pairs is incorrect?

   A. vitamin D–inhibition of cytochrome P450
   B. vitamin C–antioxidant
   C. vanillin–increase DNA repair
   D. folic acid–correct DNA methylation imbalances

368. Big Blue and Muta Mouse are examples of _____.

   A. in vitro gene mutation assays
   B. assays that test for tumor promoters and not initiators
   C. transgenic models
   D. none of the above

369. All of the following statements are true regarding gap-junctional, intracellular communication except _____.

   A. Small molecules less than 1 kDa can be exchanged through neighboring cells.
   B. It is inhibited by tumor promoters.
   C. Carcinogens that interfere with it are not tissue and species specific.
   D. It is achieved by connexin hexamers that form a pore between adjacent cells.

370. All of the following statements are true regarding GSTM1 except _____.

   A. It demonstrates high reactivity toward epoxides.
   B. Humans possessing the null isoform have a higher risk for bladder and gastric cancer.
   C. It is primarily a detoxication enzyme.
   D. The null isoform is protective in breast cancer

371. All of the following are true regarding proto-oncogenes except _____.

    A. There are no known oncogenic virus analogues.
    B. They are dominant.
    C. Somatic mutations can be activated during all stages of carcinogenesis.
    D. Germ line inheritance of these genes is rarely involved in cancer development.

372. All of the following are true regarding oncogenes except _____.

    A. no known oncogenic virus analogue.
    B. They are recessive.
    C. broad tissue specificity for cancer development
    D. somatic mutations activated during all stages of carcinogenesis

373. All of the following are true regarding tumor suppressor genes except _____.

    A. BCRA1 is an example.
    B. They are recessive.
    C. no oncogenic virus analogues
    D. Germ line inheritance is never involved in cancer development.

374. Which of the following species develops cancer after exposure to a PPAR agonist?

    A. monkey
    B. human
    C. mouse
    D. guinea pig

375. All of the following are PPAR agonists except _____.

    A. 3-methylcholanthrene
    B. clofibrate
    C. trichloroethylene
    D. diethylhexyl phthalate

376. What do PPAR alpha agonists, phenobarbital, and TCDD have in common?

   A. They all cause human cancer.
   B. They all bind to receptors that bind to response elements that modulate gene transcription.
   C. They all bind to nuclear receptors that induce cytochrome 2D6.
   D. They are all genotoxic in at least one species.

377. All of the following are agonists at the estrogen receptor in humans except _____.

   A. DES
   B. bisphenol A
   C. nonylphenol
   D. tamoxifen

378. Chemicals that increase reactive oxygen species can affect expression of genes regulating _____.

   A. proliferation
   B. differentiation
   C. apoptosis
   D. all of the above

379. Melamine causes nongenotoxic carcinogenicity by the mechanism of _____.

   A. altered-DNA methylation
   B. induction of oxidative stress
   C. cytotoxicity
   D. stimulation of PPAR alpha-receptors

380. All of the following are true of aromatic amines except _____.

   A. They are ultimate carcinogens.
   B. Aniline dyes are examples.

C. They are associated with bladder cancer.
D. They form reactive metabolites after phase 1 biotrans-formation.

381. The carcinogenicity of nongenotoxic chemicals that cause cyto-toxicity is due to _____.

A. hormonal factors
B. increase in spontaneous mutations from secondary hyperplasia
C. acidosis
D. acute phase reactants

382. All of the following produce renal tumors in male rats except _____.

A. inorganic arsenic
B. D-limonene
C. 1,4-dichlorobenzene
D. trimethylpentane

383. PPAR agonists produce all of the following tumor types in rats except _____.

A. hepatocellular carcinoma
B. pancreatic acinar cell tumors
C. Leydig cell tumors
D. glioblastoma

384. Which of the following statements is true?

A. Ethylating carcinogenic agents produce adducts mostly in the phosphate backbone of DNA.
B. Oxidative DNA adducts occur only on adenine.
C. The presence of a DNA adduct is sufficient for carcinogenesis.
D. There is no repair for oxidative DNA damage.

385. All of the following statements are true except _____.

A. The predominate adduct formed from methylating agents on DNA is 7 methyl guanine.
B. Unpaired electrons on S, O, and N are nucleophilic targets of electrophiles.
C. Hypomethylated genes are rarely transcribed.
D. Chemical carcinogens can react with proteins.

386. Which of the following carcinogen-DNA damage pairs is incorrect?

A. mustards–DNA crosslinks
B. UV light–pyrimidine dimers
C. nongenotoxic carcinogens–7 alkylguanine
D. ionizing radiation–double-stranded breaks

387. Which of the following statements is incorrect?

A. Mutations in an oncogene can result in a clonal cell population with a survival advantage.
B. DNA damage leads to cell death or neoplasms, never to synthesis of abnormal proteins.
C. Human cancer is usually the result of chronic exposure to a carcinogen.
D. DNA polymerases can correct miscopied DNA bases during replication.

388. All of the following are examples of DNA repair except _____.

A. reverse transcriptive repair
B. mismatch repair
C. excision repair
D. end-joining repair of nonhomologous DNA

389. All of the following are reactive carcinogenic electrophiles except _____.

   A. strained lactones
   B. carbonium ions
   C. selenium ion
   D. epoxides

390. Direct-acting carcinogens include all of the following except _____.

   A. mustard gases
   B. imines
   C. sulfate esters
   D. aromatic rings

391. Which of the following is an ultimate carcinogen?

   A. safrole
   B. aflatoxin B1
   C. benzidine
   D. benzo[a]pyrene 7,8-diol 9,10-epoxide

392. Which of the following is a procarcinogen?

   A. benzo[a]pyrene
   B. benzo[a]pyrene 7,8-epoxide
   C. aflatoxin B1-2,3-epoxide
   D. methyl carbonium ion

393. All of the following are true of the dominant lethal assay except _____.

   A. Males are the treated sex.
   B. Both germ cell and somatic cell mutations are measured.
   C. Embryonic death is the endpoint.
   D. The mouse or rat is usually used.

394. The first indication that a chemical is a mutagen is often its _____.

    A. pKa
    B. chemical structure
    C. octanol-water partition coefficient
    D. dielectric constant

395. Smokers are likely to have _____.

    A. increased numbers of SCE
    B. increased frequency of chromosomal aberrations
    C. increased number of DNA adducts
    D. all of the above

396. The detection of chromosome alterations has been made easier by the development of _____.

    A. FISH
    B. HERS
    C. BASH
    D. NORM

397. Mutation by chemicals usually causes all of the following except _____.

    A. DNA adducts
    B. base substitutions
    C. double stranded DNA breaks
    D. errors of DNA replication

398. Aneuploidy can be defined as _____.

    A. the gain of one or more chromosomes
    B. the loss of one or more chromosomes
    C. both A and B
    D. neither A nor B

399. All of the following statements are true except _____.

   A. About 0.01 % of newborns are afflicted with genetic diseases.
   B. About 5 % of all recognized pregnancies contain chromosomal abnormalities.
   C. The frequency of aneuploidy in human sperm is 3–4 %.
   D. About 30 % of all spontaneous abortions and fetal deaths are associated with chromosomal abnormalities.

400. All of the following statements are true regarding endogenous DNA damage except _____.

   A. DNA replication is error prone and contributes to incorrect base sequences.
   B. Endogenous agents are responsible for 3 errors per hundred cells per day.
   C. Generation of reactive oxygen species contributes to errors.
   D. Deanimation of cytosines and 5-methylcytosines contribute to errors.

401. All of the following statements are true regarding DNA repair except _____.

   A. Error-free repair restores DNA to its undamaged state.
   B. Error-prone repair restores DNA to an improved but still modified state.
   C. Certain polymerases can bypass lesions that would otherwise block replication.
   D. If DNA damage is extensive, the cell will always undergo necrosis.

402. Radiomimetic chemicals are defined as _____.

   A. those that are mutagenic to germ cells but not somatic cells.
   B. those that are mutagenic mainly in the S phase of the cell cycle.

C. those that are mutagenic to somatic cells but not germ cells.

D. those that are mutagenic in all stages of the cell cycle.

403. The battle between DNA repair and DNA replication is regulated toward the repair side by the presence of _____.

   A. H-Ras
   B. EGFR
   C. p53
   D. PGDF

404. The male germ cell that can accumulate genetic change is _____.

   A. spermatogonial stem cell
   B. spermatocyte
   C. spermatid
   D. spermatozoa

405. Which of the following statements is true?

   A. Chromosome abnormalities caused by ionizing radiation are generally caused by errors of DNA replication on a damaged DNA template.
   B. The oocyte is resistant to the formation of mutations by nonradiomimetic chemicals.
   C. The oocyte is resistant to the mutagenic effect of radiation.
   D. none of the above

406. Aneuploidy has been associated with _____.

   A. griseofulvin and colchicine
   B. amoxicillin and cephalexin
   C. methicillin and cephalothin
   D. all of the above

407. In genetic toxicity testing, the move from short-term tests to more complicated mammalian tests has an associated increase in _____ .

    A. cost
    B. time
    C. relevance to humans
    D. all of the above

408. Which of the following is true of both genotoxic and nongenotoxic carcinogens?

    A. mutagenicity
    B. no theoretical threshold
    C. Tumorigenicity is dose responsive.
    D. no direct DNA damage

409. Which of the following is a common characteristic of both the initiation and progression stages of chemical carcinogenesis?

    A. reversibility
    B. irreversibility
    C. Multiple hits are a necessity.
    D. can be genotoxic or nongenotoxic

410. All of the following are direct-acting carcinogens except _____ .

    A. sulfur mustards
    B. methyl methanesulfonate
    C. Bis (chloromethyl) ether
    D. N-nitrosoamines

411. All of the following statements are generally true of direct-acting chemical carcinogens except _____ .

    A. They are highly species specific.
    B. They test positive in the Ames test without metabolic activation.

C. They include epoxides and imines.

D. They include chemotherapeutic drugs

412. Chloroform-induced liver tumors are postulated to form via which mechanism?

A. oxidative stress

B. cytotoxicity

C. hormonal

D. receptor mediated

413. The gold standard for determining whether chemicals have the potential to cause cancer in humans is _____.

A. Ames test

B. mouse lymphoma assay

C. Chinese hamster ovary assay

D. 2-year study in laboratory rodents

414. Which of the following is true of asbestos?

A. Its association with lung cancer is greatly increased in the presence of cigarette smoking.

B. It causes only peritoneal mesothelioma.

C. It causes cancer by DNA adduct formation.

D. It is not associated with any other lung injury except neoplasms.

415. A test that has a greater than 85 % concordance with the 2-year rodent bioassay is _____.

A. in vitro prokaryote mutagenesis

B. Syrian hamster embryo

C. mouse lymphoma assay

D. Chinese hamster ovary

416. All of the following are examples of genotoxicity and not mutagenicity except _____.

    A. unscheduled DNA synthesis
    B. sister chromatal exchanges (SCE)
    C. purine transition
    D. DNA strand breaks

417. Which of the following statements is true regarding a forward mutation assay?

    A. The Ames test is an example.
    B. It has a greater than 95 % concordance with the 2-year rodent carcinogenicity test.
    C. The response is usually broader than a reverse mutation assay.
    D. It directly measures chemical adducts to DNA.

418. A membrane-bound structure that is a simple indicator of chromosome damage is_____.

    A. endoplasmic reticulum
    B. micronucleus
    C. microsome
    D. histone

419. The difference between mutagenic and genotoxic is _____.

    A. Genotoxicity only causes birth defects.
    B. Mutagenicity produces transmissible genetic alterations.
    C. Mutagenicity only refers to chemicals and not ionizing radiation.
    D. Genotoxicity produces transmissible genetic alterations.

420. Which of the following statements is true?

   A. Structure-activity relationships have been of little value in predicting mutagenesis.
   B. Nongenotoxic chemicals can be species specific.
   C. There is no statistical difference in the frequency of chromosomal aberrations between human smokers and nonsmokers.
   D. Chromosomal aberrations have not been shown to increase with age in humans.

CHAPTER 6 ANSWERS (REFERENCES)

344. C (I)	380. A (I)	416. C (III)
345. B (I)	381. B (I)	417. C (III)
346. B (I)	382. A (I)	418. B (III)
347. B (I)	383. D (I)	419. B (III)
348 . B (I)	384. A (I)	420. B (III)
349. A (I)	385. C (I)	
350. C (I)	386. C (I)	
351. C (I)	387. B (I)	
352. A (I)	388. A (I)	
353. D (I)	389. C (I)	
354. D (I)	390. D (I)	
355. A (I)	391. D (I)	
356. B (II)	392. A (I)	
357. A (II)	393. B (III)	
358. C (II)	394. B (I)	
359. D (I)	395. D (I,III)	
360. B (I)	396. A (III)	
361. A (I)	397. C (III)	
362. A (I)	398. C (III)	
363. D (I)	399. A (III)	
364. C (I)	400. B (III)	
365. B (I)	401. D (III)	
366. D (I)	402. D (III)	
367. A (I)	403. C (III)	
368. C (I)	404. A (III)	
369. C (I)	405. B (III)	
370. D (I)	406. A (III)	
371. A (I)	407. D (III)	
372. B (I)	408. C (I)	
373. D (I)	409. B (I)	
374. C (I)	410. D (I)	
375. A (I)	411. A (I)	
376. B (I)	412. B (I)	
377. D (I)	413. D (I)	
378. D (I)	414. A (I)	
379. C (I)	415. B (I)	

REFERENCES

CHAPTER 6

I.   J. E. Klaunig and L. M. Kamendulis, "Chemical Carcinogens," in *Casarett & Doull's Toxicology: The Basic Science of Poisons*, 7th ed., ed. C. D. Klaassen (New York: McGraw-Hill, 2008), 329–380.

II. G. M. Williams, M. J. Iatropoulos, and H. G. Enzmann, "Principles of Testing for Carcinogenic Activity," in *Principles and Methods of Toxicology*, 5th ed., ed. A. W. Hayes (Boca Raton: CRC Press, 2008), 1265–1316.

III. J. R. Preston and G. R. Hoffman, "Genetic Toxicology," in *Casarett & Doull's Toxicology: The Basic Science of Poisons*, 7th ed., C. D. Klaassen (New York: McGraw-Hill, 2008), 381–414.

7

TOXICOLOGY DURING DEVELOPMENT

421. The percentage of major congenital defects at birth is estimated to be _____.

    A. less than 1 %
    B. 2 to 3 %
    C. 5 to 7 %
    D. none of the above

422. All of the following antimicrobials are human developmental toxicants except _____.

    A. penicillins
    B. tetracyclines
    C. aminoglycosides
    D. fluconazole

423. All of the following metals are human developmental toxicants except _____.

    A. lithium
    B. lead
    C. organic mercury
    D. copper

424. All of the following infectious agents are human developmental toxicants except _____.

A. rubella virus
B. influenza virus
C. syphilis
D. toxoplasmosis

425. All of the following are human developmental toxicants except _____.

A. folic acid
B. ethanol
C. cocaine
D. tobacco smoke

426. The FDA protocol that primarily examines teratogenicity is _____.

A. segment I
B. segment II
C. segment III
D. segment IV

427. Which of the following statements is true regarding concordance of findings regarding developmental toxicity between animals and humans?

A. Concordance is strongest when there are positive data from more than one species treated.
B. Humans tend to be more sensitive than the most sensitive animal test species.
C. The mouse and rat tend to be better test species than the rabbit.
D. All of the above

428. In the PDR, most drugs are listed as a "use in pregnancy" category _____.

   A. A
   B. B
   C. C
   D. D

429. All of the following are true regarding the Sonic Hedgehog pathway (SHH) except _____.

   A. SHH is primarily linked to transcription of tumor-suppression genes.
   B. Ligands for SHH require covalent binding of cholesterol.
   C. Mutations of the SHH gene can cause holoprosencephaly in mice and humans.
   D. The pathway was first discovered in Drosophila.

430. The majority of congenital malformations in humans are due to _____.

   A. radiation
   B. infectious agents
   C. alcohol
   D. unknown factors

431. Potential endocrine-disrupting chemicals on the estrogen receptor include all of the following except _____.

   A. flutamide
   B. methoxychlor
   C. chlordecone
   D. phytoestrogens

432. Potential endocrine-disrupting chemicals that antagonize the androgen receptor include all of the following except _____.

   A. vinclozolin
   B. finasteride

C. bisphenol A

D. p,p'DDE

433. The FDA protocol that primarily examines fertility and preimplementation and postimplantation viability is _____.

A. segment I

B. segment II

C. segment III

D. segment IV

434. The FDA protocol that primarily examines postnatal survival, growth, and external morphology is _____.

A. segment I

B. segment II

C. segment III

D. segment IV

435. Indirect-toxicant developmental effects due to maternal toxicity include all of the following except _____.

A. cocaine's effect on uterine blood flow

B. ethanol's effect on maternal folate

C. thalidomide's effect on angiogenesis in the offspring

D. ethanol's effect on maternal zinc

436. All of the following maternal diseases have been associated with adverse pregnancy outcomes except _____.

A. allergic rhinitis

B. febrile illness during the first trimester

C. hypertension

D. diabetes mellitus

437. The incidence of neural tube defects in the offspring of pregnant women could be reduced by supplementation early in pregnancy with _____.

    A. niacin
    B. folate
    C. biotin
    D. riboflavin

438. All of the following are true of the developmental toxicity of cadmium except _____.

    A. It appears to involve placental toxicity.
    B. It appears to involve inhibition of nutrient transport across the placenta.
    C. Zinc can affect the developmental toxicity of cadmium.
    D. Cadmium induces transferrin, which binds zinc in the placenta.

439. All of the following are true regarding induction of metallothionein in pregnant rats except _____.

    A. It can be caused by urethane, ethanol, or alpha-hederin
    B. Induction is directly related to maternal zinc retention.
    C. High-dose vitamin C can prevent the induction.
    D. Induction is inversely related to zinc distribution to the offspring.

440. All of the following processes are necessary for a normally developing embryo except _____.

    A. apoptosis
    B. cell proliferation
    C. cell differentiation
    D. necrosis

441. Embryos deficient in p53 _____.

    A. transform into choriocarcinoma
    B. do not survive into organogenesis
    C. develop normally
    D. none of the above

442. All of the following statements are true regarding toxicant effects on an embryo except _____.

    A. Cellular predisposition to apoptosis can vary.
    B. The creation of a normal or malformed offspring depends on the cellular balance between damage and repair.
    C. Cellular insults to an embryo can include those affecting cell-cell interactions and energy metabolism.
    D. The developing heart is very sensitive to toxicant-induced apoptosis.

443. Advances in molecular biology that have helped understand the mechanisms involved in abnormal development are _____.

    A. cell staining and flow cytometry
    B. antisense oligonucleotides and knockout mice
    C. prion research and PCR technology
    D. all of the above

444. Which of the following statements is true?

    A. The mammalian embryo lacks P450 enzymes.
    B. The mammalian embryo has P450 activity comparable to the maternal liver.
    C. The mammalian embryo is incapable of metabolizing chemicals to active teratogens.
    D. None of the above.

445. All of the following statements are true except _____.

    A. Mammalian developmental toxicity is considered a threshold event.
    B. Angiotensin converting enzyme inhibitors are safe during the first trimester.
    C. All epileptic women are at an increased risk for birth defects.
    D. Antiepileptic medications besides valproic acid are teratogens.

446. All of the following are true of the process of imprinting except _____.

    A. It is not susceptible to toxicants.
    B. It occurs during gametogenesis.
    C. It involves cytosine methylation.
    D. It may be involved in paternally mediated developmental toxicity.

447. All of the following statements are true except _____.

    A. The blastocyst consists of about 1,000 cells; however, only a very small number eventually form the embryo.
    B. Gastrulation is the process of the formation of 3 primary germ layers.
    C. The gastrulation period is not susceptible to teratogenesis.
    D. Chemicals affecting DNA synthesis and microtubule assembly are particularly toxic during the preimplantation period.

448. The fetal period is characterized by all of the following except _____.

    A. beginning organ development
    B. tissue differentiation
    C. growth
    D. physiologic maturation

449. Toxic exposure during the fetal period is likely to cause effects on _____.

A. organogenesis
B. implantation
C. growth and maturation
D. all of the above

450. All of the following are true regarding tobacco smoke exposure during pregnancy except _____.

A. Approximately 25 % of women continue to smoke during pregnancy.
B. Nicotine is a neutroteratogen in experimental animals.
C. Gene polymorphisms may place some mothers at increased risk of adverse fetal effects.
D. Passive smoke is not a risk factor for adverse fetal effects.

451. All of the following are true regarding retinoid exposure during pregnancy except _____.

A. There is some evidence for a link to schizophrenia.
B. Vitamin A is not teratogenic.
C. The RXR alpha-receptor may play a role in cleft palate development.
D. 13-cis-retinoic acid is a marketed drug that is FDA pregnancy category X.

452. Fetal malformations have occurred after pregnant mice have had brief (approximately 6-hour) exposure immediately following fertilization to _____.

A. ethylene oxide
B. oxygen
C. methane
D. sulfur dioxide

453. The concept of fetal programming means that the maternal developmental environment _____.

    A. during the first 2 weeks of pregnancy will affect organogenesis
    B. can be manipulated to produce superior offspring
    C. can partially determine metabolic parameters in the offspring that will persist throughout life
    D. all of the above

454. When is the neural plate formed in the human body?

    A. days 15–17
    B. days 18–20
    C. days 21–24
    D. days 25–28

455. All of the following were congenital abnormalities associated with thalidomide except _____.

    A. congenital heart disease
    B. phocomelia
    C. hydrocephalus
    D. ear malformations

456. The most sensitive species for assessing thalidomide congenital abnormalities is _____.

    A. mouse
    B. human
    C. rat
    D. hamster

457. Thalidomide has been used in all of the following indications except _____.

    A. sleeping aid
    B. treatment of emphysema

C. treatment of oral ulcers in AIDS

D. treatment of erythema nodosum leprosum

458. DES was previously used in the United States to treat _____.

A. morning sickness
B. preeclampsia
C. gestational diabetes
D. threatened abortion

459. Human male offspring of DES-exposed mothers have an increased incidence of all of the following except _____.

A. low semen volume and poor semen quality
B. epididymal cysts
C. hypotrophic testes
D. prostate cancer

460. All of the following drugs are developmental toxicants except _____.

A. penicillin
B. valproic acid
C. ethanol
D. lead

461. All of the following are true of the fetal alcohol syndrome except _____.

A. craniofacial dysmorphism
B. intrauterine growth retardation
C. impaired psychomotor development
D. normal IQ

462. Maternal tobacco smoking is associated with what condition in the offspring?

A. Increased probability of twins
B. undescended testicles

C. vitiligo

D. increased risk of sudden infant death syndrome (SIDS)

463. All of the following are true of maternal cocaine exposure except
_____.

A. Fetal cocaine exposure can be estimated by chemical analysis of fetal meconium.
B. increased incidence of abruptio placentae
C. increased incidence of phocomelia
D. increased incidence microcephaly

464. Misoprostol during pregnancy can produce offspring with
_____.

A. hypothyroidism
B. situs inversis
C. limb reduction defects
D. none of the above

465. Which of the following is true of the use of angiotensin converting enzyme inhibitors during pregnancy?

A. Their effects are different from those of angiotensin receptor blockers.
B. They are associated with neonatal renal failure.
C. They adversely affect the fetus during the first trimester only.
D. They are associated with adult-onset renal cell carcinoma in the offspring.

466. The period of organogenesis in humans is _____.

A. days 21 to 56
B. days 20 to 45
C. days 15 to 32
D. days 6 to 18

467. All of the following statements are true except _____.

   A. In mammals, the formation of the neural plate signals the onset of organogenesis.
   B. Some toxicants may produce growth retardation at low doses and lethality at high doses.
   C. Gametogenesis is the process of forming the sperm and egg germ cells.
   D. Mammalian developmental toxicity has generally been considered to be a nonthreshold event.

468. All of the following are normal physiologic changes during pregnancy except _____.

   A. Cardiac output can increase by 50 %.
   B. Blood volume increases relative to red cell volume.
   C. Intestinal motility decreases.
   D. Systolic blood pressure increases.

469. Which one of the following statements is true?

   A. Most drugs cross the placenta by simple passive diffusion.
   B. There is no pH difference between the maternal and embroyonic plasma.
   C. The placentas of all mammals are very similar.
   D. The human placenta lacks drug-metabolizing enzymes.

470. Which of the following infectious agents is associated with human developmental toxicity?

   A. hepatitis C virus
   B. methicillin-resistant staph bacteria
   C. cytomegalovirus
   D. Candida albicans vaginosis

471. Approximately what percent of marketed drugs belong to FDA pregnancy category A?

    A. 1 %
    B. 10 %
    C. 20 %
    D. 30 %

Matching Test

472. indomethacin   A. spinal bifida

473. cocaine   B. staining of teeth

474. phenytoin   C. virilization of female fetus

475. ampicillin   D. neonatal hypothyroidism

476. amiodarone   E. relatively safe

477. progestins   F. premature closure of ductus arteriosus

478. valproic acid   G. fetal hydantoin syndrome

479. tetracycline   H. decreased uterine blood flow

CHAPTER 7 ANSWERS (REFERENCES)

421. B (I)
422. A (I)
423. D (I)
424. B (I)
425. A (I)
426. B (I)
427. D (I)
428. C (I)
429. A (I)
430. D (I)
431. A (I)
432. C (I)
433. A (I)
434. C (I)
435. C (I)
436. A (I)
437. B (I)
438. D (I)
439. C (I)
440. D (I)
441. C (I)
442. D (I)
443. B (I)
444. D (I)
445. B (I)
446. A (I)
447. C (I)
448. A (I)
449. C (I)
450. D (I)
451. B (I)
452. A (I)
453. C (I)
454. B (I)
455. C (I)
456. B (I)

457. B (I)
458. D (I)
459. D (I)
460. A (I)
461. D (I)
462. D (I)
463. C (I)
464. C (II)
465. B (I)
466. A (I)
467. D (I)
468. D (I)
469. A (I)
470. C (I)
471. A (I)
472. F (II)
473. H (II)
474. G (II)
475. E (II)
476. D (II)
477. C (II)
478. A (II)
479. B (II)

REFERENCES

CHAPTER 7

I. J. M. Rogers and R. L. Kavlock, "Developmental Toxicology," in *Casarett & Doull's Toxicology: The Basic Science of Poisons*, 7th ed., C. D. Klaassen (New York: McGraw-Hill, 2008), 415–454.

II. J. S. Fine, "Reproductive and Perinatal Principles," in *Goldfrank's Toxicologic Emergencies*, 9th ed., ed. L. S. Nelson et al. (New York: McGraw-Hill, 2011), 423–446.

8

IMMUNE SYSTEM TOXICOLOGY

480. All of the following are components of tertiary lymphoid tissue except _____.

    A. spleen
    B. Peyer's patches
    C. skin-associated lymphoid tissue (SALT)
    D. nasal-associated lymphoid tissue (NALT)

481. The lymphoid precursor cell is derived from _____.

    A. null cell
    B. pluripotent stem cell
    C. myeloid precursor
    D. monocyte

482. All of the following are considered nonself by the immune system except _____.

    A. cancers
    B. red blood cells
    C. bacteria
    D. viruses

483. T cell precursors are programmed to leave the bone marrow and migrate to the _____.

   A. spleen
   B. lymph nodes
   C. thymus
   D. Peyer's patches

484. Thymic education means that T cells _____.

   A. are converted to B cells
   B. are taught to recognize self versus nonself
   C. are taught to produce immunoglobulins
   D. are taught to proliferate rapidly

485. Peyer's patches _____.

   A. collect antigens from the gastrointestinal tract
   B. are parts of the tonsillar tissue
   C. are located in the center of the spleen
   D. are located in the lung

486. Tertiary lymphoid tissues _____.

   A. produce totipotent stem cells
   B. include the thymus
   C. have direct contact with the external environment
   D. all of the above

487. All of the following are parts of the innate immune system except _____.

   A. macrophages
   B. B cells
   C. NK cells
   D. polymorphonuclear cells (PMN)

488. All of the following are true of IgG except _____.

    A. It crosses the placenta.
    B. There are subclasses.
    C. It can fix complement.
    D. It can degranulate mast cells.

489. All of the following are true of IFN-α except _____.

    A. It is classified as an immunosuppressant.
    B. It is used to treat hepatitis C.
    C. It is associated with autoimmune disease.
    D. It has antiviral properties.

490. All of the following are true of antigens except _____.

    A. They are 10kDa or larger.
    B. They are nonself substances that can be recognized by the immune system.
    C. Parts of the human body can never be antigens.
    D. They can be foreign DNA, RNA, protein, or carbohydrates.

491. The inability of self-reactive T cells that escape negative selection to proliferate in response to self-antigen exposure is called _____.

    A. autoimmunity
    B. self-tolerance
    C. hypersensitivity
    D. opsonization

492. All of the following statements are true regarding developmental immunology except _____.

    A. Immune system development is complete at birth.
    B. The immune system develops from a population of pluripotent stem cells.

C. Animals with short gestation periods have relatively immature immune systems at birth compared to humans.
D. Exposure to specific antigens during the prenatal period allows the organism not to develop autoimmune reactions later in life.

493. All of the following are autoimmune diseases except _____.

A. rheumatoid arthritis
B. multiple sclerosis
C. schizophrenia
D. myasthenia gravis

494. An assay that was developed to test the immunostimulating capacity of pharmaceuticals is _____.

A. ELISA
B. flow cytometric analysis
C. popliteal lymph node assay
D. all of the above

495. All of the following are direct mechanisms of xenobiotic-induced immune modulation except _____.

A. increased mineralocorticoid release from adrenal gland
B. altered antibody-mediated response
C. altered cell-mediated response
D. altered host resistance

496. A prolonged inflammatory response may contribute to the development of _____.

A. Alzheimer's disease
B. cardiovascular disease
C. multiple sclerosis
D. all of the above

497. When a cytotoxic cell attaches to an Fc protein of IgG directed against a foreign antigen, the hypersensitivity reaction is called type _____.

A. I
B. II
C. III
D. IV

498. When IgG or IgM directed against soluble antigens produces antigen-antibody complexes that are deposited in tissues, the hypersensitivity reaction is called type _____.

A. I
B. II
C. III
D. IV

499. When an antigen processing cell interacts with T cells leading to the generation and proliferation of memory T cells, the hypersensitivity reaction is called type _____.

A. I
B. II
C. III
D. IV

500. The process of negative selection for self-reactive T cells occurs in the _____.

A. bone marrow
B. spleen
C. thymus
D. lymph nodes

501. An essential component of antigen processing is _____.

   A. return of antigen-processing cell to bone marrow
   B. a time interval of 7 days between internalization of antigen and its appearance on the cell surface
   C. binding of complement to antigen-processing cell
   D. association of modified antigen with major histocompatibility complex

502. All of the following are true except _____.

   A. Monocytes circulate in the blood for about a day.
   B. Natural killer cells (NK) are derived from the monocyte.
   C. Perforin and granzyme are mediators of cell death by natural killer cells.
   D. Polymorphonuclear cells combat microorganisms by the release of reactive oxygen species.

503. Mononuclear phagocytic cells within the central nervous system are called _____.

   A. microglia
   B. Kupffer cells
   C. stellate cells
   D. astrocytes

504. All of the following are involved in the humoral response except _____.

   A. B cell
   B. T cell
   C. eosinophil
   D. antigen-processing cell

505. In cell-mediated cytotoxicity, the target cell is induced by the effector cell to undergo _____.

   A. necrosis
   B. apoptosis

C. proliferation

D. hyperplasia

506. All of the following are true of the innate response except
_____.

A. It is less specific than acquired immunity.
B. Complement is a soluble mediator.
C. The response can be enhanced by repeated antigen exposure.
D. Acute-phase proteins are involved.

507. A substance that must be attached to a carrier molecule to elicit an immune response is called a/an _____.

A. adjunct
B. initiator
C. hapten
D. protoantigen

508. All of the following are true of the complement system except
_____.

A. It functions to destroy membranes of infectious agents and promote an inflammatory response.
B. There is no interaction with the acquired immune system.
C. Three pathways have been identified.
D. Activation occurs when components sequentially act on others.

509. The Fc region of an antibody mediates all of the following functions except _____.

A. complement activation
B. binding to phagocytes
C. binding to leukocytes
D. inhibiting hyaluronidase of bacteria

510. All of the following are antigen-processing cells except _____.

   A. basophil
   B. macrophage
   C. follicular dendritic cell
   D. Langerhans dendritic cell

511. Individuals with low to moderate suppression of immune function are more susceptible to infections with _____.

   A. protozoans
   B. Candida albicans
   C. influenza
   D. Pneumocystis carinii

512. All of the following are true regarding the immunotoxicology of halogenated aromatic hydrocarbons except _____.

   A. They are particularly immunotoxic in mice.
   B. They are associated with thymic atrophy in animal models.
   C. Their effects are mediated through AHR.
   D. Prolonged human exposure can result in death from immunodeficiency.

513. Which of the following toxicant-reaction pairs is incorrect?

   A. benzopyrene–metabolized by bone marrow
   B. TCDD-chloracne
   C. PCDF–recurring respiratory infections
   D. PBB–severe human immunodeficiency

514. All of the following statements are true except _____.

   A. Malathion demonstrates both immune suppression and immune enhancement.
   B. The immunotoxicity of organophosphates is due to suppression of acetylcholinesterase.

C. Parathion suppresses both cell-mediated and humoral immunity.
D. There is a correlation between DDE levels in breast milk and infant ear infections.

515. All of the following can suppress the immune system except _____.

A. zinc
B. arsenic
C. lead
D. mercury

516. Which of the following statements is true regarding opioid use and HIV infection?

A. Morphine increases CCR5 expression.
B. Heroin use is associated with increased risk of HIV infection.
C. Opioid use may contribute to HIV progression through immune suppression.
D. All of the above

517. All of the following have been associated with increased risk for development of scleroderma in at least one clinical study except _____.

A. cocaine
B. silica
C. vinyl chloride
D. organic solvents

518. All of the following gases have been shown to alter pulmonary immunologic response except _____.

A. ozone
B. carbon dioxide
C. sulfur dioxide
D. nitrogen dioxide

519. All of the following metals (not salts) are associated with a high incidence of contact dermatitis except _____.

    A. chromium
    B. nickel
    C. platinum
    D. colbalt

520. Hypersensitivity to latex can be manifested in all of the following ways except _____.

    A. pulmonary fibrosis
    B. asthma
    C. urticaria
    D. anaphylaxis

521. Papain and subtilin are _____.

    A. mold toxins
    B. mushroom toxins
    C. commercial enzymes
    D. hypersensitivity agents in latex

522. All of the following statements are true except _____.

    A. Risk assessment in immunotoxicology is a highly accurate exercise.
    B. Many chemicals can alter the immune system of animals.
    C. Perturbations in immune function can occur in the absence of any clinically observable effect.
    D. Alterations in immune function are correlated with an increased risk of infectious diseases.

523. The Buehler test is used to assess _____.

    A. autoimmunity
    B. pulmonary hypersensitivity
    C. type III hypersensitivity reactions
    D. contact hypersensitivity

524. Respiratory sensitization in animals is primarily an indication of a/an _____.

    A. type I reaction
    B. type II reaction
    C. type III reaction
    D. autoimmune reaction

525. A xenobiotic that enhances immune function is called _____.

    A. promoter
    B. hapten
    C. regulator
    D. adjuvant

526. The overall immunocompetence of an individual is affected least by _____.

    A. hair color
    B. age
    C. gender
    D. nutritional status

527. In general, acute-phase reactants are associated with _____.

    A. regulating the clotting system
    B. binding toxicants for renal excretion
    C. downregulation of the immune system
    D. induction of drug metabolism

528. Natural killer cells have surface markers that are similar to _____.

    A. B cells
    B. T cells
    C. neither B or T cells
    D. both B and T cells

529. The most common type of immune modulation that occurs from exposure to xenobiotics is _____.

   A. automimmune disease
   B. hypersensitivity
   C. carcinogenesis
   D. lymphadenopathy

530. The immunotoxicity of PCBs, PCDFs, and PCDDs is thought to occur by _____.

   A. binding to the glucocorticoid receptor
   B. binding to the estrogen receptor
   C. binding to the aryl hydrocarbon receptor
   D. binding to the androgen receptor

531. The gender-related differences in human immune function include all of the following except _____.

   A. Males have higher levels of circulating immunoglobulins.
   B. Females have a greater antibody response.
   C. Females have a higher incidence of autoimmune disease.
   D. Males are more susceptible to the development of sepsis.

532. A potent inhibitor of protein synthesis is found in _____.

   A. snake venom toxin
   B. black widow spider toxin
   C. black mold toxin
   D. oleander plant toxin

533. Besides their effects on secondary sex characteristics, estrogens are also associated with _____.

   A. dental caries protection
   B. enhanced wound healing
   C. decreased gastric acid secretion
   D. anti-inflammatory effects

534. Which of the following is associated with immunosuppression in humans?

A. opioids
B. cannabinoids
C. ethanol
D. all of the above

535. The major concern with genetically modified food crops is _____.

A. production of electrophiles leading to carcinogenesis
B. expression of novel proteins that could be recognized as nonself by the immune system
C. decrease in nutritional value
D. modification of natural bacterial flora in small and large intestine

536. All of the following are associated with a systemic lupus erythematosus-like syndrome except _____.

A. procainamide
B. hydralazine
C. isoniazid
D. methyldopa

537. Halothane hepatitis is _____.

A. automimmune
B. cholestatic
C. vascular
D. none of the above

538. Xenobiotic-induced system lupus erythematosus is an example of _____.

A. autoimmunity
B. hypersensitivity

C. immunostimulation

D. immunosuppression

539. Toluene diisocyanate commonly causes _____.

A. autoimmunity

B. hypersensitivity

C. immunostimulation

D. immunosuppression

540. Azathioprine commonly causes _____.

A. autoimmunity

B. hypersensitivity

C. immunostimulation

D. immunosupression

Matching Test

541. IgM

A. T cell surface marker

542. NK cells

B. contributes to hyperalgesia

543. IgA

C. noncellular component of innate immunity

544. IL-1

D. primary lymphoid tissue

545. GM-CSF

E. secretory antibody

546. CD8

F. derived from myeloid precursor cell

547. IgE

G. causes fever

548. prostaglandins

H. derived from bone marrow stem cells

549. megakaryocyte

I. stimulates growth/differentiation of granulocyte

550. bone marrow

J. possibly involved in pathogenesis of asthma

551. coughing

K. antibody that peaks before IgG

CHAPTER 8 ANSWERS (REFERENCES)

480. A (I)	516. D (I)
481. B (I)	517. A (I)
482. B (I)	518. B (I)
483. C (I)	519. C (I)
484. B (I)	520. A (I)
485. A (I)	521. C (I)
486. C (I)	522. A. (I)
487. B (I)	523. D (I)
488. D (I)	524. A (I)
489. A (I)	525. D (I)
490. C (I)	526. A (I)
491. B (I)	527. C (I)
492. A (I)	528. C (I)
493. C (I)	529. B (I)
494. C (I)	530. C (I)
495. A (I)	531. A (I)
496. D (I)	532. C (I)
497. B (I)	533. D (I)
498. C (I)	534. D (I)
499. D (I)	535. B (I)
500. C (I)	536. D (I)
501. D (I)	537. A (I)
502. B (I)	538. A (I)
503. A (I)	539. B (I)
504. C (I)	540. D (I)
505. B (I)	541. K (I)
506. C (I)	542. H (I)
507. C (I)	543. E (I)
508. B (I)	544. G (I)
509. D (I)	545. I (I)
510. A (I)	546. A (I)
511. C (I)	547. J (I)
512. D (I)	548. B (I)
513. D (I)	549. F (I)
514. B (I)	550. D (I)
515. A (I)	551. C (I)

REFERENCE

CHAPTER 8

I.   N. E. Kaminski, B. L. Faubert Kaplan, and M. P. Holsapple, "Toxic Responses of the Immune System," in *Casarett & Doull's Toxicology: The Basic Science of Poisons*, 7th ed., C. D. Klaassen (New York: McGraw-Hill, 2008), 485–556.

9

HEMATOLOGIC TOXICOLOGY

552. All of the following statements are true regarding hematopoiesis except _____.

   A. In children it is confined to the yellow or fatty marrow.
   B. In adults, it is confined to the axial skeleton and proximal humerus and femur.
   C. Under extreme conditions, embryonic patterns may reoccur.
   D. The bone marrow is the only blood cell producing organ at birth.

553. All of the following could be features of megaloblastic anemia except _____.

   A. low serum B12 or folate
   B. microcytosis (decreased MCV)
   C. pancytopenia
   D. hypersegmented neutrophils

554. All of the following are associated with megaloblastic anemia except _____.

   A. phenytoin
   B. ethanol
   C. aspirin
   D. methotrexate

555. All of the following are characteristics of aplastic anemia except
_____.

A. causation by radiation exposure
B. peripheral blood pancytopenia
C. bone marrow hypoplasia
D. reticulocytosis

556. All of the following have been associated with aplastic anemia
except _____.

A. gold
B. chloramphenicol
C. acetone
D. felbamate

557. A defect in the synthesis of the porphyrin ring of heme can
produce _____.

A. iron precipitation within mitochondria
B. sideroblastic anemia
C. accumulation of iron in bone marrow
D. all of the above

558. All of the following are true of carboxyhemoglobin except
_____.

A. Low concentrations can be cytoprotectice during
inflammatory stress.
B. Symptoms appear at levels of 3 %.
C. The oxygen-disassociation curve is shifted to the left.
D. Smoking during pregnancy could produce levels in the fetus
that decrease tissue oxygenation.

559. Methemoglobin can reversibly bind all of the following ions
except _____.

A. calcium
B. azide

C. sulfide

D. cyanide

560. Infectious diseases causing direct hemolysis of red blood cells include all of the following except _____.

A. malaria

B. babesiosis

C. chlamydial urethritis

D. bartonellosis

561. During oxidative hemolysis of red blood cells, the ferric iron in heme can react with chloride to form a complex called _____.

A. Heinz bodies

B. hemin

C. hemosiderin

D. beta 2 microglobin

562. The major enzymes that protect against oxidative injury in red blood cells include all of the following except _____.

A. aldehyde reductase

B. superoxide dismutase

C. glutathione peroxidase

D. NADH-diaphorase

563. All of the following have been associated with oxidative injury to red blood cells except _____.

A. primaquine

B. ethanol

C. dapsone

D. nitrofurantoin

564. Snake venom produces _____.

A. oxidative hemolytic anemia

B. nonoxidative chemical-induced hemolytic anemia

C. immune hemolytic anemia
D. all of the above

565. All of the following are mechanisms for drug-induced immune hemolytic anemia except _____.

A. hapten
B. conformational change in erythrocyte membrane
C. schistocyte formation
D. drug-induced autoantibody

566. An enzyme that markedly increases in the serum after hemolysis is _____.

A. alkaline phosphatase
B. creatine phosphokinase
C. acid phosphatase
D. lactic dehydrogenase

567. Eosinophilia is seen in all of the following conditions except _____.

A. toxic oil syndrome
B. contaminated tryptophan preparations
C. megaloblastic anemia
D. drug allergic reactions

568. All of the following are true of neutrophils except _____.

A. a "shift to the right" occurs during major infection
B. Serious infections can occur when counts fall lower than 500 per microliter.
C. G-CSF regulates both neutrophil production and release from the bone marrow.
D. Bands and metamyelocytes are immature forms that can appear in the peripheral blood during infection.

569. An inhibition of CXR-chemokine ligand and CXCR4 will be expected to _____.

    A. mobilize stem cells from the bone marrow
    B. mobilize mature neutrophils from the bone marrow
    C. treat the myelotoxicity of cancer chemotherapy
    D. all of the above

570. Which of the following is most likely to cause neutropenia?

    A. lithium carbonate
    B. lindane
    C. dexamethasone
    D. hydrocortisone

571. All of the following inhibit phagocytosis except _____.

    A. glucocorticoids
    B. ethanol
    C. iohexol
    D. calcium ion

572. All of the following are true regarding idiosyncratic toxic neutropenia except _____.

    A. It may or may not be dose related.
    B. Toxicants that do not affect uncommitted stem cells are associated with a better outcome.
    C. It usually persists for months after drug withdrawal.
    D. The immunologic form is more common in women and the elderly.

573. All of the following agents affect stem cells except _____.

    A. aminopyrine
    B. gold
    C. chloramphenicol
    D. phenylbutazone

574. Which of the following is true for clozapine-induced agranulocytosis?

    A. The incidence, even with frequent monitoring, is 6 %.
    B. A genetic predisposition has been established.
    C. Olanzapine causes agranulocytosis by the same mechanism.
    D. all of the above

575. All of the following are true of immune neutropenia except _____.

    A. The incidence is considerably higher than immune hemolytic anemia.
    B. Direct antigranulocyte antibodies are difficult to measure.
    C. Antigen-antibody reactions can lead to the destruction of peripheral neutrophils, granulocyte precursors, or both.
    D. Propylthiouracil causes neutropenia by this mechanism.

576. Deletions in chromosomes 5 and 7 occur at a low frequency in _____.

    A. AML secondary to alkalating agents
    B. AML secondary to benzene
    C. AML secondary to topoisomerase II inhibitors
    D. Nontoxicant and nonchemotherapy-related AML

577. The two conditions most frequently associated with drug or chemical exposure are _____.

    A. AML and CLL
    B. AML and ALL
    C. AML and MDS
    D. AML and CML

578. Current theories on the origin of AML suggest _____.

    A. It is a multievent progression.
    B. It is caused by an infectious RNA virus.
    C. In utero exposure to a toxicant is necessary for development.
    D. none of the above

579. For which of the following drugs is causation data for AML inconclusive?

    A. cyclophosamide
    B. busulfan
    C. chlorambucil
    D. none of the above

580. There is considerable evidence that xylene causes _____.

    A. CLL
    B. CML
    C. ALL
    D. None of the above

581. All of the following are associated with heparin-induced thrombocytopenia except _____.

    A. formation of an immune complex that binds to platelets
    B. retroperitoneal hematomas
    C. arterial thrombosis
    D. venous thrombosis

582. Thrombotic thrombocytopenic purpura (TTP) has been associated with all of the following except _____.

    A. cocaine
    B. hydrochlorothiazide
    C. ticlopidine
    D. clopidogrel

583. All of the following are associated with an increased risk of bleeding except _____.

    A. aspirin
    B. ibuprofen
    C. vitamin B6
    D. N-methylthiotetrazole cephalosporins

584. All of the following will decrease bleeding except _____.

    A. nadolol
    B. aprotinin
    C. aminocaproic acid
    D. tranexamic acid

585. All of the following are true of lupus anticoagulants except _____.

    A. They are antibodies that interfere with phospholipid-dependent coagulation reactions.
    B. They potentiate procoagulant mechanisms.
    C. They can cause severe bleeding.
    D. They can be induced by procainamide and hydralazine.

586. All of the following are true of heparin except _____.

    A. Unfractionated heparin causes a higher incidence of thrombocytopenia.
    B. It causes osteoporosis.
    C. It crosses the placenta.
    D. It causes transaminase elevations.

587. To detect one adverse event in a clinical trial that occurs at a frequency of 1 % at a 95 % confidence level, how many test subjects need to be exposed?

    A. 100
    B. 300
    C. 500
    D. 1000

588. A hematologic problem detected through postmarketing surveillance was _____.

    A. bleeding and urokinase
    B. acute allergy and streptokinase
    C. aplastic anemia and felbamate
    D. leukopenia and tranexamic acid

589. A grading system for hematologic toxicity was established in 1979 by _____.

A. WHO
B. FDA
C. EPA
D. OSHA

590. Serial blood and bone marrow sampling is best done in _____.

A. hamster
B. rat
C. dog
D. mouse

591. All of the following are advantages of in vitro bone marrow assays except _____.

A. can examine effects on myeloid, erythroid, and platelet precursors
B. can predict pharmacokinetics in humans
C. can examine combination of chemicals
D. can make interspecies comparisons

592. A chemical causing nonoxidative chemical-induced hemolysis of red blood cells is _____.

A. hydrogen sulfide
B. arsine
C. ozone
D. xylene

593. Drug-induced immunohemolytic anemia is associated with all of the following except _____.

A. alpha-methyldopa
B. warfarin
C. penicillin
D. quinidine

594. The hemolytic uremic syndrome has been linked to _____.

    A. endotoxin-producing Pseudomonas aeruginosa
    B. tetradotoxin
    C. emetic toxins from B. cerus
    D. verocytotoxin from E. coli

595. Acetaminophen overdosage would first affect the clotting factor with the shortest half-life, which would be _____.

    A. II
    B. VII
    C. IX
    D. X

596. All of the following have been associated with warfarin except _____.

    A. hepatitis
    B. congenital abnormalities
    C. bone demineralization
    D. skin necrosis

597. All of the following are true regarding methemoglobin except _____.

    A. Methylene blue is not an effective antidote in G6PD deficiency.
    B. The predominant detoxication pathway involves methemoglobin reductase and NADPH.
    C. Most patients tolerate low levels (< 10 %) of methemoglobin without clinical symptoms.
    D. Aniline dyes are causative agents.

598. The hemoglobin-oxygen dissociation curve is shifted to the left by _____.

    A. fever
    B. acidosis

C. hypophosphatemia

D. 2,3-BPG

599. The presence of schistocytes on a peripheral blood smear is indicative of _____.

A. iron deficiency

B. lead poisoning

C. malaria

D. microangiopathic hemolytic anemia

600. Oxidative injury to red blood cells is most severe in humans with a deficiency of _____.

A. glucose-6-phosphate dehydrogenase

B. cytochrome P450 2E1

C. aspartate transaminase

D. creatine phosphokinase

601. In the human fetus, hematopoiesis can occur in all of the following organs except _____.

A. liver

B. lung

C. spleen

D. thymus

602. An imbalance in the production of alpha and beta globulin chains is the basis for _____.

A. iron deficiency anemias

B. congenital thalassemia syndromes

C. sideroblastic anemias

D. megaloblastic anemia

603. Ringed sideroblasts are characteristic of anemias caused by
_____.

A. alpha methyldopa
B. phenytoin
C. lead
D. folate deficiency

604. Pure red cell aplasia is caused by all of the following except
_____.

A. isoniazid
B. acetaminophen
C. phenytoin
D. azathioprine

Matching Test

605. desmopressin   A. megaloblastic anemia

606. mitomycin   B. left shift of hemoglobin-oxygen
                                   curve

607. quinidine   C. bleeding

608. lead   D. microcytic anemia

609. triamterene   E. hemolytic anemia and
                                   thrombocytopenia

610. aromatic benzaldehydes   F. treatment of von Willebrand's
                                   disease

611. dicumarol   G. hemolytic uremic syndrome

CHAPTER 9 ANSWERS (REFERENCES)

552. A (I)	588. C (I)
553. B (I)	589. A (I)
554. C (I)	590. C (I)
555. D (I)	591. B (I)
556. C (I)	592. B (I)
557. D (I)	593. B (I)
558. B (I)	594. D (I)
559. A (I)	595. B (I)
560. C (I)	596. A (I)
561. B (I)	597. B (I)
562. A (I)	598. C (I)
563. B (I)	599. D (I)
564. B (I)	600. A (I)
565. C (I)	601. B (I)
566. D (I)	602. B (I)
567. C (I)	603. C (I)
568. A (I)	604. B (I)
569. D (I)	605. F (I)
570. B (I)	606. G (I)
571. D (I)	607. E (I)
572. C (I)	608. D (I)
573. A (I)	609. A (I)
574. B (I)	610. B (I)
575. A (I)	611. C (I)
576. D (I)	
577. C (I)	
578. A (I)	
579. D (I)	
580. D (I)	
581. B (I)	
582. B (I)	
583. C (I)	
584. A (I)	
585. C (I)	
586. C (I)	
587. B (I)	

REFERENCE

CHAPTER 9

I.   J. C. Bloom and J. T. Brandt, "Toxic Responses of the Blood," in *Casarett & Doull's Toxicology: The Basic Science of Poisons*, 7th ed., ed. C. D. Klaassen (New York: McGraw-Hill, 2008), 455–484.

10

HEPATIC TOXICOLOGY

612. Early stages of ethanol abuse are characterized by _____.

   A. inability to degrade lipids in the liver
   B. inability to transport lipids out of the liver
   C. increased lipid synthesis within the liver
   D. all of the above

613. The liver is the first organ to encounter all of the following except _____.

   A. waste products of bacteria in the gut
   B. inhaled gases
   C. ingested metals
   D. oral drugs

614. Zone 3 of the hepatic acinus is characterized by _____.

   A. high bile acid concentrations
   B. relative hypoxia
   C. proximity to the portal vein
   D. proximity to the hepatic artery

615. Zone 1 of the hepatic acinus is characterized by _____.

   A. high levels of glutathione
   B. higher levels of P450

C. proximity to the hepatic vein

D. low bile acid extraction

616. CYP 2E1 is highest in acinus zone _____.

    A. 1

    B. 2

    C. 3

    D. 4

617. Decreased protein synthesis by the liver would cause all of the following conditions except _____.

    A. ascites

    B. hypoglycemia

    C. bleeding

    D. increased free fraction of drugs

618. All of the following are components of bile except _____.

    A. glutathione

    B. cholesterol

    C. uric acid

    D. bilirubin

619. Bile acid formation plays a key role in all of the following processes except _____.

    A. the innate immune system

    B. excretion of endogenous compounds

    C. uptake of lipid nutrients from the small intestine

    D. protection of the small intestine from oxidative insult

620. Rats lacking a functional MRP2 biliary exporter would be expected to be resistant to the _____.

    A. fibrosis from ethanol

    B. intestinal ulceration from diclofenac

C. carcinogenicity of androgens
D. fatty liver from tamoxifen

621. A major site for vitamin A storage is _____.

A. hepatocyte
B. cholangiocyte
C. Kupffer cell
D. stellate cell

622. Hepatic sinusoids are lined with all of the following cells except _____.

A. stellate cells
B. endothelial cells
C. Kupffer cells
D. enterocytes

623. All of the following statements are true of hepatic fenestrae except _____.

A. Molecules smaller than 250 kDa can cross.
B. Albumin can cross.
C. The space between hepatocyte and endothelium in which molecules cross the fenestrae is known as the space of Disse.
D. They are similar to the pores in skeletal muscle.

624. Which one of the following statements is true?

A. The liver cannot regenerate.
B. Methylmercury is reabsorbed from the gallbladder.
C. Zinc toxicity is manifested by cholestasis.
D. all of the above

625. A transport pump that moves chemicals from hepatocyte into bile caniculi is _____.

A. OAT
B. BSEP

C. OCT

D. all of the above

626. Which one of the following statements is true?

A. Arsenic is enterohepatically recirculated.

B. Microcystin disrupts the hepatic cytoskeleton.

C. Biliary epithelial cells possess biotransformation enzymes.

D. all of the above

627. The most common cause of fatty liver is _____.

A. valproic acid

B. fialuridine

C. insulin resistance

D. carbon tetrachloride

628. All of the following statements are true regarding steatosis and steatohepatitis except _____.

A. Cycloheximide causes fat accumulation and cell necrosis.

B. Steatohepatitis can progress to fibrosis.

C. The presence of steatosis can make a liver more sensitive to ischemia or other toxins.

D. Steatohepatitis can progress to hepatocellular carcinoma.

629. Dilation of the hepatic sinusoid or peliosis hepatis is caused by _____.

A. amiodarone

B. danazol

C. tetracycline

D. halothane

630. Vanishing bile duct syndrome is associated with all of the following except _____.

A. ethanol

B. carbamazepine

C. anabolic steroids

D. contraceptive steroids

631. All of the following have been shown to inhibit the bile salt export pump (BSEP) except _____.

A. rifampicin

B. bosentan

C. troglitazone

D. acetaminophen

632. In the liver, the difference between oncotic necrosis and secondary necrosis is _____.

A. cell swelling

B. cell content release

C. identification of many apoptotic cells

D. none of the above

633. A pancaspase inhibitor would be expected to _____.

A. prevent apoptosis-induced liver injury in isolated hepatocytes

B. induce oncotic liver cell necrosis

C. deplete cellular ATP by damaging the mitochondrial membrane

D. none of the above

634. Vitamin C causes _____.

A. fatty liver

B. canalicular cholestasis

C. bile duct damage

D. none of the above

635. Drug-induced steatosis is mainly caused by compounds that _____.

A. accumulate in lysozymes and breakdown cellular lipids

B. accumulate in mitochondria and inhibit beta-oxidation

C. accumulate in cytosol and stimulate lipid synthesis

D. none of the above

636. Bile duct and gallbladder cancer is increased in individuals exposed to _____.

   A. phenacetin
   B. bromobenzene
   C. vinyl chloride
   D. radioactive thorium dioxide

637. All of the following statements are true regarding hepatocellular carcinoma except _____.

   A. Malignant transformation can result from increased cell turnover due to chronic injury and persistent inflammation.
   B. DNA modifications can lead to activation of cellular oncogenes.
   C. The cancer cells are highly sensitive to alkylating chemotherapy.
   D. Stimulation of proliferation leads to expansion of preneoplastic cells prior to neoplastic transformation.

638. Central to the development of fibrosis is _____.

   A. activation of hepatic stellate cells
   B. suppression of Kupffer cells
   C. stimulation of an antibody response
   D. formation of DNA adducts

639. All of the following are true regarding hepatic fibrosis except _____.

   A. Stimulation of apoptosis in causative cells may lead to a gradual reversal.
   B. It is caused by increased membrane collagen type IV.
   C. It can interfere with the exchange of nutrients and waste material between hepatocyte and sinusoidal blood.
   D. Viral hepatitis is the primary cause of hepatic fibrosis/ cirrhosis worldwide.

640. Iron overload causes preferential damage in _____.

    A. zone 1 hepatocytes
    B. zone 2 hepatocytes
    C. zone 3 hepatocytes
    D. zone 4 hepatocytes

641. Methylene dianiline is preferentially toxic to _____.

    A. hepatocytes
    B. stellate cells
    C. Kupffer cells
    D. bile duct cells

642. Cadmium hepatotoxicity is related to _____.

    A. valence of cadmium ion
    B. induction of CYP2E1
    C. saturation of hepatocyte's ability to sequester cadmium ion
       complex with metallothionein
    D. low-serum iron

643. The hepatic toxicity of acetaminophen is enhanced by all of the
     following except _____.

    A. malnutrition
    B. fasting
    C. induction of CYP2E1
    D. hypertension

644. Steatosis from chronic alcohol consumption is thought to result
     from _____.

    A. stimulation of beta-oxidation of fatty acids
    B. excess supply of acetate and NADH
    C. excess supply of pyruvate and NADP+
    D. inhibitory effect of acetaldehyde on fatty acid breakdown

645. Which of the following is thought to be an important factor in the pathology of alcohol-induced liver disease?

    A. inflammatory response
    B. lipid peroxidation
    C. oxidative stress
    D. all of the above

646. Allyl alcohol is metabolized by ADH to _____.

    A. benzaldehyde
    B. acrolein
    C. acetic anhydride
    D. butyraldehyde

647. Endotoxin and GdCl$_3$ preferentially activate _____.

    A. stellate cells
    B. Kupffer cells
    C. zone 3 hepatocytes
    D. bile duct cells

648. Most of a therapeutic dose of acetaminophen is _____.

    A. metabolized to NAPQI
    B. acetylated
    C. conjugated with glycine
    D. none of the above

649. Which of the following expresses the recent thinking with respect to neutrophils and liver damage?

    A. Detrimental liver effects can occur from neutrophil mobilization to other organs.
    B. Injury occurs by the killing of distressed cells that would otherwise survive.

    C. Neutrophils participate in the same way in all types of toxic liver injury.

    D. Damage is exacerbated by the mass killing of healthy liver cells.

650. All of the following cause nonimmune idiosyncratic liver toxicity except _____.

    A. tienilic acid
    B. isoniazid
    C. amiodarone
    D. ketoconazole

651. All of the following statements are true regarding idiosyncratic drug-induced hepatoxicity except _____.

    A. It probably involves failure to adapt to a mild drug adverse effect combined with a genetic defect.
    B. Traditional animal toxicology studies may not detect it.
    C. Carbon tetrachloride is an example.
    D. Preclinical studies may need to be done in genetically deficient animals to detect some examples.

652. Ethyl alcohol is metabolized in humans by all of the following except _____.

    A. CYP3A4
    B. CYP2E1
    C. ADH
    D. peroxisomal catalase

653. All of the following hepatic sites are matched with the appropriate preferential toxicant except _____.

    A. zone 1 hepatocyte–iron
    B. bile duct cells–ethanol
    C. stellate cells–vitamin A
    D. zone 3 hepatocyte–carbon tetrachloride

654. All of the following are true regarding ethanol and the liver except _____.

    A. Ethanol inhibits the transfer of triglycerides from liver to adipose tissue.
    B. Alcohol dehydrogenase is the only inducible enzyme in chronic alcoholics.
    C. An inactive form of aldehyde dehydrogenase is found in 50 % of Asians.
    D. The catalase pathway is a minor route for ethanol metabolism.

655. All of the following are true regarding the hepatoxicity of carbon tetrachloride except _____.

    A. The reactive metabolite is formed by cytochrome P450 3A4.
    B. The reactive metabolite is a free radical.
    C. Chronic ethanol exposure can enhance the injury.
    D. The injury involves lipid peroxidation.

656. Idiosyncratic liver injury is characterized by all of the following except _____.

    A. can be immune or nonimmune mediated
    B. has a clear dose-response relationship
    C. is relatively rare
    D. has a probable genetic basis

657. Wilson's disease is due to _____.

    A. increased intestinal absorption of copper
    B. decreased biliary excretion of copper
    C. decreased renal excretion of copper
    D. increased sensitivity to normal levels of copper

658. The liver cell process associated with cell swelling, leakage of cell contents, and an influx of inflammatory cells is _____.

  A. apoptosis
  B. fibrosis
  C. necrosis
  D. steatosis

659. Fatty liver is caused by all of the following except_____.

  A. ethanol
  B. vinyl chloride
  C. carbon tetrachloride
  D. insulin resistance

660. Which cell is located in the Space of Disse?

  A. stellate cell
  B. endothelial cell
  C. Kupffer cell
  D. bile duct cells

661. Heptacellular carcinoma is associated with all of the following except _____.

  A. doxycycline
  B. aflatoxin
  C. viral hepatitis
  D. androgen abuse

Matching Test

662. albumin

663. aspartate transaminase

664. prothrombin time

665. ammonia

666. alkaline phosphatase

667. ultrasound

668. gamma glutamyl transpeptidase

669. bilirubin

A. elevated in liver disease and hemolysis

B. elevated in liver and bone disease

C. decreased in chronic liver disease

D. elevated in 60-80 % of patients with hepatic encephalopathy

E. most sensitive indicator of acute liver disease

F. distinguishes bone from liver disease

G. demonstrates extrahepatic bile duct dilation

H. reflects level of coagulation factors

CHAPTER 10 ANSWERS (REFERENCES)

612. B (I)	648. D (I)
613. B (I)	649. B (I)
614. B (I)	650. A (I)
615. A (I)	651. C (I)
616. C (I)	652. A (I)
617. B (I)	653. B (I)
618. C (I)	654. B (I)
619. A (I)	655. A (I)
620. B (I)	656. B (I)
621. D (I)	657. B (I)
622. D (I)	658. C (I)
623. D (I)	659. B (I)
624. B (I)	660. A (I)
625. B (I)	661. A (I)
626. D (I)	662. C (II)
627. C (I)	663. E. (II)
628. A (I)	664. H (II)
629. B (I)	665. D (II)
630. A (I)	666. B (II)
631. D (I)	667. G (II)
632. C (I)	668. F (II)
633. A (I)	669. A (II)
634. D (I)	
635. B (I)	
636. D (I)	
637. C (I)	
638. A (I)	
639. B (I)	
640. A (I)	
641. D (I)	
642. C (I)	
643. D (I)	
644. B (I)	
645. D (I)	
646. B (I)	
647. B (I)	

REFERENCES

CHAPTER 10

I. H. Jaeschke, "Toxic Responses of the Liver," in *Casarett & Doull's Toxicology: The Basic Science of Poisons*, 7th ed., ed. C. D. Klaassen (New York: McGraw-Hill, 2008), 557–582.

II. K. A. Delaney, "Hepatic Principles," in *Goldfrank's Toxicologic Emergencies*, 9th ed., ed. L. S. Nelson et al. (New York: McGraw-Hill, 2011), 367–380.

11

RENAL TOXICOLOGY

670. The kidney is involved in all of the following metabolic processes except _____.

   A. phase 1 biotransformation
   B. synthesis of aldosterone
   C. synthesis of renin
   D. synthesis of erythropoietin

671. A toxicant transported to the kidney via the blood will have the highest delivery rate to the renal _____.

   A. medulla
   B. cortex
   C. papilla
   D. none of the above

672. Which of the following is least likely to pass through the glomerulus?

   A. polycationic macromolecules
   B. inulin
   C. polyanionic macromolecules
   D. neutral macromolecules

673. The portion of the proximal tubule that is characterized by a tall brush border and a well-developed vascular lysosomal system is _____.

    A. S1
    B. S2
    C. S3
    D. S4

674. The portion of the proximal tubule that is noted for catabolism, high apical transport of glutathione, and high gamma-glutamyl transpeptidase is _____.

    A. S1
    B. S2
    C. S3
    D. S4

675. Analgesic nephropathy is due to the long-term use of the combination of _____.

    A. NSAIDs and acetaminophen
    B. acetaminophen and opiates
    C. opiates and NSAIDs
    D. tramadol and acetaminophen

676. NSAID use is associated with _____.

    A. renal allograph rejection
    B. interstitial nephritis
    C. renal cell carcinoma
    D. all of the above

677. A process that plays a role in aminoglycoside proximal tubule nephrotoxicity is _____.

    A. deposition of immune complexes
    B. free radical formation

C. decrease in intracellular calcium

D. phopholipidosis

678. A process that plays a key role in the nephrotoxicity of halogenated hydrocarbons is _____.

A. selective transport

B. tubular secretion

C. renal vasoconstrictor

D. biotransformation

679. One mechanism for the renal toxicity of cyclosporin is thought to be increased production of _____.

A. thromboxane

B. vasodilatory prostaglandins

C. endorphins

D. aldosterone

680. In the presence of superoxide anion, nitric oxide can be converted into which of the following agents implicated in renal ischemia/ reperfusion injury?

A. nitric oxide radical

B. nitrogen anion

C. peroxynitrite anion

D. nitrogen dioxide anion

681. If a nephrotoxicant's primary mechanism of action is ATP depletion, _____.

A. Apoptosis will dominate oncosis at all toxicant concentration.

B. Oncosis may be the main cause of cell death, with limited apoptosis occurring.

C. Oncosis will never occur.

D. none of the above

682. A test to measure renal blood flow in humans is _____.

    A. insulin clearance
    B. creatinine clearance
    C. serum cystatin C
    D. none of the above

683. Binding to renal sulfhydryl groups is thought to play a role in the renal toxicity of _____.

    A. metals
    B. fluoride ion
    C. aminoglycocides
    D. hydrogen sulfide

684. An increase in urinary excretions of alkaline phosphatase and gamma glutamyl transpeptidase suggests damage to _____.

    A. glomerules
    B. collecting duct
    C. afferent anteriole
    D. brush border

685. A drug that interacts with sterols and causes the distill tubular epithelium to leak water and ions is _____.

    A. methoyflurane
    B. amphotericin B
    C. fentanyl
    D. acetaminophen

686. A test to evaluate glucosuria in the presence of a normal serum glucose would be _____.

    A. urine pH
    B. 24-hour excretion of albumin
    C. 24-hour excretion of B_2 microglobulin
    D. urine creatinine

687. A characteristic of renal glomerular injury is _____.

   A. albuminuria
   B. white cell casts
   C. uric acid crystals on urinalysis
   D. amino acids in the urine

688. Serum creatinine is not a very sensitive indicator of renal function because _____.

   A. It is increased in liver disease.
   B. About 50 % of renal function has to be lost before it will rise.
   C. It decreases with exercise.
   D. all of the above

689. BUN can be increased in all of the following except _____.

   A. dehydration
   B. hypovolemia
   C. protein catabolism
   D. immediately postdialysis

690. ACE inhibitors will most likely precipitate acute renal failure in patients with _____.

   A. congestive heart failure
   B. systolic hypertension
   C. bilateral renal artery stenosis
   D. mitral stenosis

691. Immune complexes characteristically cause injury to the _____.

   A. proximal tubule
   B. loop of Henle
   C. glomerulus
   D. collecting duct

692. Changes in charge selectivity of the renal glomerulus secondary to toxicants are due to _____.

    A. decrease in positively charged sites
    B. decrease in negatively charged sites
    C. increase in positively charged sites
    D. increase in negatively charged sites

693. All of the following are important in the selective proximal tubular toxicity of many toxicants except _____.

    A. plasma level of bilirubin
    B. cellular level of CYP450
    C. cellular level of cysteine B-lyase
    D. selective cellular transport

694. Ischemic injury to the proximal tubule can be precipitated by toxicants that interfere with all of the following except _____.

    A. permeability of the collecting duct to water
    B. renal blood flow
    C. cellular energetics
    D. mitochondrial function

695. A compensatory response to renal injury that may be maladaptive over time is _____.

    A. increased vasopressin secretion
    B. decreased renin secretion
    C. decreased renal blood flow
    D. increase in glomerular pressure

696. Factors that are presumed to play a role in the pathogenesis of chronic renal failure include all of the following except _____.

    A. growth factor promoters and inhibitors
    B. DNA-adduct formation

C. lipid accumulation

D. extracellular matrix deposition

697. The kidney is susceptible to toxic injury for all of the following reasons except _____.

A. The processes involved in forming dilute urine are also involved in concentrating toxicants in tubular fluid.

B. Any toxicant in the systemic circulation will be delivered to the kidney.

C. A nontoxic concentration of a toxicant in the circulation can reach toxic concentrations in the kidney.

D. Insoluble chemicals may precipitate out and cause tubular obstruction.

698. High-circulating concentrations of renal vasoconstrictor hormones are normally counterbalanced by _____.

A. thromboxane

B. prostaglandins

C. aldosterone

D. vasopressin

699. All of the following mechanisms can decrease GFR except _____.

A. increased glomerular hydrostatic pressure

B. afferent arteriolar constriction

C. back leakage of glomerular filtrate

D. obstructing tubular casts

700. Following toxic damage to the kidney, casts obstructing the tubular lumen are composed primarily of _____.

A. neutrophils and macrophages

B. red cells and white cells

C. basophils and plasma cells

D. necrotic and viable tubular cells

701. Following a toxic insult to tubular epithelial cells, the reparative and adaptive response is believed to be derived primarily from _____.

   A. bone marrow-derived stem cells
   B. surviving tubular epithelial cells
   C. dedifferentiated capillary endothelial cells
   D. migration and redifferentiation of adrenal cortical cells

702. As a compensatory process, uninjured renal cells following nephrotoxic exposure can undergo all of the following except _____.

   A. hypertrophy
   B. apoptosis
   C. adaptation
   D. proliferation

703. Cellular adaptation responses to toxicant-induced renal injury include the induction of all of the following except _____.

   A. metallothionein
   B. heat shock proteins
   C. glucose-regulated proteins
   D. BRCA1

704. In a normal healthy individual, a substance that is filtered by the kidney and completely reabsorbed without any excretion is _____.

   A. creatinine
   B. urea
   C. glucose
   D. sodium

705. The portion of the nephron with a high Na+/K+ATPase activity and low oxygen supply is the _____.

    A. glomerulus
    B. medullary-thick ascending limb of the loop of Henle
    C. S3 segment of proximal tubule
    D. collecting duct

706. Agents that interfere with vasopressin synthesis, secretion, or action can impair which of the following the most?

    A. glomerular filtration
    B. renal bicarbonate excretion
    C. renal sodium excretion
    D. renal concentrating ability

707. Prerenal factors that can cause a decrease in GFR include all of the following except _____.

    A. glomerulonephritis
    B. congestive heart failure
    C. dehydration
    D. pre-glomerular vasoconstriction

708. Postrenal factors that can cause a decrease in GFR include all of the following except _____.

    A. ureter calculi
    B. renal tubular cell injury
    C. extrinsic ureter compression
    D. bladder outlet obstruction

709. The toxicity cisplatin is thought to be due to _____.

    A. the release of ammonia
    B. the plutonium atom
    C. its conversion to the trans isomer
    D. the geometry of the complex or a metabolite

710. A radiocontrast agent with a low incidence of nephrotoxicity would have which of the following properties?

    A. nonionic at physiologic pH
    B. high osmolarity
    C. presence of iodine
    D. high protein binding

711. Principal cells and intercalated cells are located in a 2:1 ratio in the _____.

    A. proximal tubule
    B. cortical collecting duct
    C. loop of Henle
    D. distal tubule

712. The juxtaglomerular apparatus is involved in the secretion of _____.

    A. angiotensin 1
    B. aldosterone
    C. renin
    D. vitamin D

713. The most common site of renal injury is the _____.

    A. glomerulus
    B. proximal tubule
    C. loop of Henle
    D. collecting duct

714. Which of the following is true of the mercuric ion?

    A. It is more neurotoxic than organic mercury.
    B. It preferentially binds to amino groups over sulfhydryl groups.
    C. Chelation therapy is of no benefit in the nephrotoxicity of the mercuric ion.
    D. The S3 segment of the proximal tubule is the initial site of toxicity.

715. All of the following are true of the renal glomerulus except
_____.

A. Twenty percent of blood flow entering the glomerulus is filtered.
B. Filtration of cationic molecules are restricted more than anionic.
C. Toxicants can affect the charge barrier and allow for the urinary excretion of formally restricted molecules.
D. Filtration of macromolecules is generally inversely proportional to molecular weight.

716. Which of the following is the correct toxicant-target organ pair?

A. penicillamine-glomerulus
B. immune complexes–collecting duct
C. analgesic mixtures–proximal tubule
D. heavy metals–loop of Henle

CHAPTER 11 ANSWERS (REFERENCES)

670. B (I)
671. B (I)
672. C (I)
673. A (I)
674. C (I)
675. A (I)
676. B (I)
677. D (I)
678. D (I)
679. A (I)
680. C (I)
681. B (I)
682. D (I)
683. A (I)
684. D (I)
685. B (I)
686. C (I)
687. A (II)
688. B (I)
689. D (I)
690. C (I)
691. C (I)
692. B (I)
693. A (I)
694. A (I)
695. D (I)
696. B (I)
697. A (I)
698. B (I)
699. A (I)
700. D (I)
701. B (I)
702. B (I)
703. D (I)
704. C (I)
705. B (I)

706. D (I)
707. A (II)
708. B (II)
709. D (I)
710. A (I)
711. B (III)
712. C (III)
713. B (I)
714. D (I)
715. B (I)
716. A (I)

REFERENCES

CHAPTER 11

I.   R. G. Schnellmann, "Toxic Responses of the Kidney," in *Casarett & Doull's Toxicology:Tthe Basic Science of Poisons*, 7th ed., ed. C. D. Klaassen (New York: McGraw-Hill, 2008), 583–608.

II.   D. A. Feinfeld and N. B. Harbord, "Renal Principles," in *Goldfrank's Toxicologic Emergencies*, 9th ed. L. S. Nelson et al. (New York: McGraw-Hill, 2011), 381–395.

III. L. H. Lash, "Principles and Methods for Renal Toxicology," in *Principles and Methods of Toxicology*, 5th ed., ed. A. W. Hayes (Boca Raton: CRC Press, 2008), 1509–1540.

12

CARDIOVASCULAR TOXICOLOGY

717. What is the resting potential of a cardiac myocyte relative to extracellular fluid?

    A. -120 to -90mV
    B. -90 to -60 mV
    C. -60 to -30 mV
    D. -30 to -10 mV

718. All of the following positive ions are involved in the bioelectricity of the heart except _____.

    A. Mg+2
    B. Na+1
    C. K+1
    D. Ca+2

719. The phase of the action potential during which there is rapid inward movement of sodium ion is called phase _____.

    A. 0
    B. 1
    C. 2
    D. 3

720. The sinus node pacemaker cells and Purkinje fibers in the ventricles are examples of cardiac cells that have the property of _____.

    A. dedifferentiation
    B. phagocytosis
    C. automaticity
    D. six phases of the action potential

721. Excitation-contraction coupling requires all of the following except _____.

    A. entry of extracellular calcium into the cell
    B. hydrolysis of ATP
    C. a conformational change in the cardiac myocyte thin filament
    D. binding of calcium to acid phosphatase

722. Contraction and relaxation of individual cardiac myocytes in an organized manner to perform efficient pump function is achieved by _____.

    A. neurohormonal regulation
    B. neurotransmitter release
    C. electronic cell-to-cell coupling
    D. local release of cytokines

723. The QRS segment of the electrocardiograph represents _____.

    A. atrial depolarization
    B. conduction time through the ventricles
    C. ventricular repolarization
    D. B and C

724. A normal ST segment is _____.

    A. biphasic
    B. elevated 2–3 mm from baseline
    C. depressed 2–3 mm from baseline
    D. none of the above

725. Which of the following molecules is responsible for the largest energy stores in the heart?

    A. ATP
    B. creatine
    C. phosphocreatine
    D. ADP

726. During toxicant-induced damage to cardiac mitochondria, there is an energy shift to reliance on _____.

    A. oxidation of free fatty acids
    B. deamination of amino acids
    C. ATP produced in the liver
    D. anaerobic glucose metabolism

727. All of the following are cellular events causing cardiomyopathy from toxicant exposure except _____.

    A. myocardial cell death
    B. myocyte hyperplasia
    C. extracellular matrix remodeling
    D. apoptosis

728. Which of the following is associated with heart hypertrophy rather than heart failure after toxicant exposure?

    A. fetal gene expression
    B. apoptosis
    C. dilation
    D. all of the above

729. Factors that can convert cardiac hypertrophy into cardiac failure include all of the following except _____.

    A. ANP
    B. ET-1
    C. TNF
    D. angiotensin II inhibitors

730. Lethal cardiac arrhythmia has been associated with _____.

    A. maladaptive cardiac hypertrophy
    B. QT prolongation
    C. myocardial infarction
    D. all of the above

731. A recent discovery that challenges the concept of the permanent loss of cardiac myocytes following cell death is the identification of _____.

    A. cardiac progenitor cells
    B. cytokines that inhibit apoptosis
    C. growth factors that stimulate hypertrophy
    D. cytokines that stimulate angiogenesis

732. A prolonged QTc interval in humans is considered greater than _____.

    A. 400 ms
    B. 420 ms
    C. 460 ms
    D. 500 ms

733. All of the following can prolong the QT interval except _____.

    A. genetic polymorphisms
    B. class III antiarrhythmics
    C. hyperkalemia
    D. exposure to particulate matter air pollution

734. A biomarker for inflammation that may predict future cardiac events in asymptomatic individuals is _____.

    A. CK-MM
    B. myoglobin
    C. BNP
    D. C-reactive protein

735. One theory for arrhythmia secondary to cardiac hypertrophy is
_____.

    A. unbalanced distribution of Purkinje fibers in the remodeling
heart
    B. increase in intracellular magnesium in hypertrophied cells
    C. increase in systemic blood pressure secondary to increased
cardiac output
    D. none of the above

736. Besides alterations in potassium channels, long QT syndrome
could result from dysfunction in _____.

    A. sodium channels
    B. chloride channels
    C. glutamate channels
    D. GABA channels

737. At the cellular level, many toxicants cause cardiac toxicity by
_____.

    A. increasing intracellular pH
    B. decreasing intracellular calcium
    C. stabilizing cardiac myocyte membranes
    D. increasing intracellular calcium

738. Hypertrophic growth of cardiac myocytes involves the activation
of _____.

    A. calcineurin
    B. thromboxane
    C. retinoic acid receptor
    D. all of the above

739. One mechanism for anthracycline cardiac toxicity is _____.

    A. stimulation of salt and water retention
    B. inhibition of myocyte apoptosis

C. stimulation of myocyte apoptosis

D. inhibition of angiogenesis

740. All of the following are involved in cardiac toxic responses except _____.

A. BCRP

B. AMPK

C. MAPK

D. PKC

741. An index that correlates with the severity of heart failure is _____.

A. C-reactive protein

B. urinary excretion of cyclic AMP

C. myocardial phosphocreatine /ATP ratio

D. total LDH

742. Myocardial degenerative responses to toxic insult include all of the following except _____.

A. myocardial cell death

B. fibrosis

C. hyperplasia

D. contractile dysfunction

743. In addition to toxic effects on cardiac myocytes, toxicants can cause cardiac toxicity by affecting _____.

A. the AHR receptor

B. angiogenesis

C. the corticosteroid receptor

D. all of the above

744. Which of the following is associated with pathological hypertrophy of the heart?

A. hypertension

B. exercise

C. pregnancy
D. none of the above

745. Myocardial accumulation of collagen is not associated with
_____.

   A. ischemic cardiomyopathy
   B. myocardial infarction
   C. pathological hypertrophy
   D. adaptive hypertrophy

746. At the molecular level, cardiac myocyte hypertrophy is associated
with _____.

   A. inhibition of tumor necrosis factor
   B. stimulation of p53
   C. reintroduction of the fetal gene program
   D. ligand binding to the androgen receptor

747. Counterregulatory factors involved in the progression of heart
hypertrophy to heart failure include all of the following except
_____.

   A. oxytocin
   B. BNP
   C. ANP
   D. TNF alpha

748. Counterregulatory mechanisms in response to compensatory
mechanisms to cardiac hypertrophy lead to _____.

   A. decrease in heart size
   B. myocardial remodeling
   C. decrease in cardiac fibrosis
   D. decrease in salt/water retention

749. During xenobiotic-induced progression to heart failure, the inflammatory cytokine TNF-alpha stimulates _____.

A. QT interval shortening
B. upregulation of hyperplastic genes
C. apoptosis
D. increased renal fractional excretion of sodium

750. Moxifloxacin is associated with _____.

A. acute congestive heart failure
B. prolongation of the QT interval
C. coronary artery thrombotic events
D. toxic cardiomyopathy

751. COX-2 inhibitors presumably increase the risk for cardiovascular events by causing _____.

A. heart block
B. systolic dysfunction heart failure
C. toxic cardiomyopathy
D. coronary artery thrombotic events

752. Inflammatory lesions in the vascular system are termed _____.

A. vasculitis
B. embolitis
C. thrombitis
D. angioinflammation

753. The most prevalent vascular structural injury is _____.

A. capillary hyperplasia
B. varicose veins
C. angioma
D. atherosclerosis

754. Elevation of serum levels of endothelin-1 is a marker for _____.

  A. cardiac myxoma in humans
  B. heart failure in humans
  C. QT interval shortening in humans
  D. fetal cardiac abnormalities during third trimester pregnancy

755. Which of the following is false regarding the heart?

  A. Cardiac hypertrophy during growth is a normal physiologic process.
  B. Cardiac myocytes make up less than half of all the cells in the heart.
  C. Congestive heart failure is associated with an increase in number of cardiac myocytes.
  D. Cardiac fibroblasts make up approximately 90 % of nonmyocyte cells.

756. Which of the following is true regarding the heart?

  A. Under normal conditions, glucose provides most of the energy demand.
  B. In CHF, there is a shift from glucose to fatty acid energy supply.
  C. Toxicants can impair oxidative phosphorylation and lead to anaerobic metabolism.
  D. Creatine is made in the heart.

757. Which of the following is true regarding the heart in myocardial infarction?

  A. Aspartate transaminase is the most sensitive marker of myocardial damage.
  B. Apoptosis does not play a part.
  C. Myocytes undergo rapid cell division.
  D. none of the above

758. A key event in initiation of apoptosis in the heart is the release of _____.

    A. cytochrome c
    B. sodium
    C. creatine
    D. none of the above

759. Which of the following is true of mitochondrial DNA?

    A. It is exposed to less oxidative injury than nuclear DNA.
    B. It is protected by histones.
    C. It has a more efficient DNA repair mechanism than nuclear DNA.
    D. Damage to it may be involved in the cardiac toxicity of doxorubicin.

760. A factor in whether a cell undergoes apoptosis or necrosis is _____.

    A. ATP concentration
    B. beta-2 microglobulin concentration
    C. amyloid A concentration
    D. C-reactive protein concentration

761. All of the following are true of adaptive and maladaptive cardiac hypertrophy except _____.

    A. Both are associated with cardiac myocyte hypertrophy.
    B. Both are associated with accumulation of collagen.
    C. Maladaptive hypertrophy increases the risk for serious arrhythmias.
    D. Adaptive hypertrophy occurs after exercise.

762. A risk factor for the development of torsade de pointes is _____.

    A. hyperkalemia
    B. hypernatremia

C. prolonged QT interval

D. all of the above

763. Which of the following toxicant-effect pairs is incorrect?

A. carbon disulfide–atherogenic in lab animals

B. nicotine–Alzheimer's disease

C. cadmium-hypertension

D. tobacco smoke–endothelial injury

764. All of the following are true of alcoholic cardiomyopathy except
_____.

A. It is unrelated to the duration of alcohol exposure.

B. Acetaldehyde may be involved in the genesis.

C. Multiple factors such as malnutrition, beverage additives, and cigarette smoking have been implicated.

D. Alcohol has been implicated as causing up to 40 % of nonischemic, dilated cardiomyopathy.

765. Which of the following is true of class 1 antiarrhythmic drugs?

A. They include lidocaine, quinidine, and flecanide.

B. They are sodium channel blockers.

C. They have proarrhythmic effects in patients with a past history of myocardial infarction.

D. all of the above

766. Sotalol is _____.

A. a beta-blocker and alpha-blocker

B. a beta-blocker and class III antiarrhythmic

C. a class I and class III antiarrhythmic

D. a beta-blocker and class IV antiarrhythmic

767. Class III antiarrhythmics are primarily _____.

A. sodium channel blockers

B. potassium channel blockers

    C. chloride channel blockers

    D. beta-adrenergic blockers

768. Cardiac glycosides like digoxin _____.

    A. increase the sensitivity of myocytes to calcium

    B. inhibit sodium/potassium ATPase

    C. cause sinus tachycardia

    D. inhibit sympathetic outflow at high doses

769. Which of the following is the most sensitive clinical indicator of myocardial cell damage?

    A. urine CPK

    B. serum troponin

    C. serum ALT

    D. serum creatinine

770. Which of the following is an indicator of fluid overload in congestive heart failure?

    A. urine pH

    B. serum CPK

    C. brain naturetic peptide (BNP)

    D. first-degree AV block on ECG

Matching Test

771. oral contraceptives

A. metal associated with essential hypertension

772. homocysteine

B. cardiac hemangiosarcomas in lab animals

773. beta-amyloid

C. abortions and abruption placentae

774. carbon disulfide

D. noncirrhotic portal hypertension in humans

775. mercury

E. increased risk of thrombotic events in users who smoke

776. particulate matter

F. preglomerular vasoconstriction and disruption of blood-brain barrier

777. arsenic

G. Elevated serum levels are associated with increased risk of atherosclerosis and venous thrombosis.

778. cocaine

H. associated with increased cardiovascular and respiratory morbidity and mortality

779. lead

I. may contribute to Alzheimer's disease

780. 1,3-butadiene

J. endothelial damage and hypothyroidism

781. hydrazinobenzoic acid

K. smooth muscle tumors in mice

CHAPTER 12 ANSWERS (REFERENCES)

717. B (I)
718. A (I)
719. A (I)
720. C (I)
721. D (I)
722. C (I)
723. B (I)
724. D (I)
725. C (I)
726. D (I)
727. B (I)
728. A (I)
729. D (I)
730. D (I)
731. A (I)
732. C (I)
733. C (I)
734. D (I)
735. A (I)
736. A (I)
737. D (I)
738. A (I)
739. C (I)
740. A (I)
741. C (I)
742. C (I)
743. B (I)
744. A (I)
745. D (I)
746. C (I)
747. A (I)
748. B (I)
749. C (I)
750. B (I)
751. D (I)
752. A (I)

753. D (I)
754. B (I)
755. C (I)
756. C (I)
757. D (I)
758. A (I)
759. D (I)
760. A (I)
761. B (I)
762. C (I)
763. B (I)
764. A (I)
765. D (I)
766. B (I)
767. B (I)
768. B (I)
769. B (I)
770. C (I)
771. E (I)
772. G (I)
773. I (I)
774. J (I)
775. F (I)
776. H (I)
777. D (I)
778. C (I)
779. A (I)
780. B (I)
781. K (I)

REFERENCE

CHAPTER 12

I.   Y. J. Kang, "Toxic Responses of the Heart and Vascular System," in *Casarett & Doull's Toxicology: The Basic Science of Poisons*, 7th ed., ed. C. D. Klaassen (New York: McGraw-Hill, 2008), 699–739.

13

DERMAL TOXICOLOGY

782. Which of the following can compromise the stratum corneum barrier and lead to increased penetration of chemicals?

   A. tape stripping
   B. psoriasis
   C. acetone exposure
   D. all of the above

783. Which of the following statements is true?

   A. The rate of penetration of chemicals across the stratum corneum will always be a first-order process.
   B. Skin uptake of airborne chemicals is common for hydrophilic agents.
   C. Psoriasis is a disease of slow skin cell turnover.
   D. none of the above

784. Which of the following skin areas has the highest permeability?

   A. eyelids
   B. palms
   C. soles of feet
   D. forehead

785. All of the following are true regarding absorption through the epidermal appendages except _____.

    A. Chemicals can bypass the stratum corneum by this route.
    B. It is more relevant for chronic rather than acute situations.
    C. It is usually neglected for most chemicals because of the smaller relative surface compared to the stratum corneum.
    D. In some cases like benzopyrene, absorption through appendages can be primary.

786. Which of the following agents has the highest skin penetration under normal conditions?

    A. hydrophilic chemicals of high molecular weight
    B. hydrophobic chemicals of high molecular weight
    C. hydrophilic chemicals of low molecular weight
    D. hydrophobic chemicals of low molecular weight

787. All of the following are advantages of transdermal drug delivery except _____.

    A. a steady infusion rate over long-time intervals
    B. variation of infusion rate with body temperature
    C. avoiding first-pass effects
    D. preventing exposure to stomach acid

788. Which of the following statements is true regarding systemic exposure through the skin while swimming in chemically contaminated water?

    A. Exposure can occur for some chemicals.
    B. Significant exposure can only occur by swallowing the water.
    C. Significant exposure can only occur through the nasal mucous.
    D. There are no reported cases of significant human exposure by this route.

789. Eighty percent of eczema dermatitis occurs on the _____.

   A. face
   B. scalp
   C. hand
   D. chest

790. Common features of both irritant and allergic contact dermatitis include all of the following except _____.

   A. inflammatory components
   B. distinguishing biopsy characteristics
   C. vesiculation
   D. erythema

791. All of the following are true of irritant-contact dermatitis except _____.

   A. The reaction can theoretically occur in anyone if the exposure is long enough or the concentration high enough.
   B. It can sometimes resemble a second-degree burn.
   C. It requires the participation of regional lymph nodes.
   D. Sensitivity to irritants can have large variations between individuals.

792. Granulomatous disease of the skin has been shown to occur during exposure to _____.

   A. tattoo dyes
   B. beryllium
   C. zirconium compounds
   D. all of the above

793. All of the following are phototoxic drugs/chemicals except _____.

   A. ampicillin
   B. tetracycline

C. anthracene

D. 8-methoxypsoralen

794. All of the following are true of ultraviolet B (UVB) radiation except _____.

A. It induces more erythema in human compared to UVA.
B. It has been implicated in melanoma development.
C. Its intensity at the earth's surface is ten times that of UVA.
D. It is responsible for most of the tanning response.

795. The occupation with the lowest incidence of contact urticaria is _____.

A. food handler
B. office workers
C. latex glove users
D. plant and wood handlers

796. The area of the body with the thickest skin is _____.

A. forehead
B. fingertip
C. back
D. abdomen

797. Which of the following body site statements is false?

A. palms—good physical barrier
B. eyelids—sensitivity to irritants
C. axillae—moist, occluded area
D. soles—poor barrier function

798. Which of the following statements is true regarding a third-degree chemical burn?

A. The damage does not need to have a primary inflammatory component.
B. Immediate coagulative necrosis may occur.

C. Necrotic tissue can act as a chemical reservoir, with systemic absorption.
D. all of the above

799. All of the following are true regarding skin patch drug delivery except _____.

A. It is ideal for drugs with short half-lives.
B. It is very safe because drug delivery stops once the patch is removed.
C. It allows drugs to avoid first-pass metabolism.
D. Marketed skin patch drugs include nicotine, clonidine, and fentanyl.

800. All of the following are true of irritant-contact dermatitis except _____.

A. It accounts for approximately 20 % of all contact dermatitis.
B. It arises from the direct action of a chemical on the skin.
C. The response is usually proportional to the dose.
D. It can occur from repeated exposure to mild irritants.

801. Allergic-contact dermatitis is characterized by _____.

A. a B cell–mediated hypersensitivity
B. processing of antigen by the melanocyte
C. a latency period
D. all of the above

802. Incidents in Seveso, Italy, and Taiwan produced outbreaks of _____.

A. chloracne
B. malignant melanoma
C. urticaria
D. phototoxic dermatitis

803. A direct release of histamine without production of antibodies can be caused by _____.

   A. thiazide diuretics
   B. opiate analgesics
   C. tetracycline antibiotics
   D. tricyclic antidepressants

804. A drug-induced, life-threatening skin reaction that may result from apoptosis due to stimulation of death receptor pathways is _____.

   A. anaphylaxis
   B. psoriasis
   C. toxic epidermal necrolysis
   D. xeroderma pigmentation

805. Psoralens are associated with _____.

   A. acne
   B. squamous cell carcinoma
   C. phototoxic dermatitis
   D. photoallergic dermatitis

806. Arsenic is associated with _____.

   A. acne
   B. skin carcinoma
   C. phototoxic dermatitis
   D. photoallergic dermatitis

807. Beneficial effects of ultraviolet radiation include all of the following except _____.

   A. production of vitamin D
   B. treatment of elevated bilirubin in infants
   C. treatment of psoriasis with psoralens
   D. treatment of basal cell carcinoma

808. A common contact allergen is _____.

    A. iron
    B. aluminum
    C. cellulose
    D. none of the above

809. Sulfonamides can cross react in allergic-contact sensitization with _____.

    A. para-aminobenzoic acid
    B. phenyl-ethyl ether
    C. propylene glycol
    D. tetracycline

810. The contact sensitizer in poison ivy is _____.

    A. nitrobenzene
    B. pentadecylcatechol
    C. propionic acid
    D. methyl benzoate

811. All of the following are true of the skin except _____.

    A. Phase 1 and phase 2 drug-metabolizing enzymes are present.
    B. There are significant interspecies differences in toxicant absorption.
    C. Active transport takes place in the stratum corneum.
    D. Cells in the stratum corneum have lost their nucleus.

Matching Test

812. androgens   A. contact dermatitis

813. selenium   B. fixed drug eruption

814. neomycin sulfate   C. alopecia

815. barbiturates   D. nail changes

816. tetracycline   E. causes acne

817. arsenic   F. photosensitivity reaction

CHAPTER 13 ANSWERS (REFERENCES)

782. D (I)
783. D (I)
784. A (I)
785. B (I)
786. D (I)
787. B (I)
788. A (I)
789. C (I)
790. B (I)
791. C (I)
792. D (I)
793. A (I)
794. C (I)
795. B (I)
796. B (II)
797. D (I)
798. D (I)
799. B (I)
800. A (I)
801. C (I)
802. A (I)
803. B (I)
804. C (I)
805. C (I)
806. B (I)
807. D (I)
808. D (I)
809. A (I)
810. B (I)
811. C (I)
812. E (II)
813. C (II)
814. A (II)
815. B (II)
816. F (II)
817. D (II)

REFERENCES

CHAPTER 13

I.   R. H. Rice and T. M. Mauro, "Toxic Responses of the Skin," in *Casarett & Doull's Toxicology: the Basic Science of Poisons*, 7th ed., ed. C. D. Klaassen (New York: McGraw-Hill, 2008), 741–762.

II.   N. A. Lewin and L. S. Nelson, "Denmatologic Principles," in *Goldfrank's Toxicologic Emergencies*, 9th ed., ed. L. S. Nelsond et al. (New York: McGraw-Hill, 2011), 410–422.

14

NEUROTOXICOLOGY

818. When the neuronal cell body is lethally injured, the process is called _____.

    A. neuritis
    B. neuralgia
    C. axonopathy
    D. neuronopathy

819. The slowest component of axonal transport involves movement of the _____.

    A. mitochondria
    B. proteins in vesicles
    C. cytoskeleton
    D. none of the above

820. To satisfy its high energy requirements, the brain relies on _____.

    A. fatty acid oxidation
    B. aerobic glycolysis
    C. phosphocreatine
    D. anaerobic glucose metabolism

821. A purpose of circumventricular organs in the brain is to _____.

    A. allow nutrients to rapidly enter the brain
    B. actively transport xenobiotics back into the blood

C. allow for neuronal hypertrophy in response to injury

D. respond to changes in blood hormone levels

822. The high energy requirement of neuronal tissue is due to _____.

A. maintenance and reestablishment of ion gradients
B. high levels of protein synthesis and degradation
C. high level of immune surveillance
D. all of the above

823. Tardive dyskinesia is caused by long-term use of _____.

A. tricyclic antidepressants
B. phenothiazines
C. amphetamines
D. cocaine

824. An advantage that the developing nervous system has over the adult nervous system is _____.

A. less sensitivity to toxic insult
B. faster recovery from toxic insult
C. a tighter blood-brain barrier
D. none of the above

825. All of the following are associated with neuronopathies except _____.

A. cyanide
B. organic mercury
C. doxorubicin
D. gold

826. The neurotoxicity of aminoglycoside antibiotics is manifested as _____.

A. hearing loss
B. visual field deficits

C. cognitive dysfunction
D. peripheral neuropathy

827. Encephalopathy after acute exposure and peripheral neuropathy after chronic exposure has been associated with _____.

A. methanol
B. phenytoin
C. arsenic
D. 6-aminonicotinamide

828. Encephalopathy has been associated with all of the following except _____.

A. streptomycin
B. lead
C. aluminum
D. carbon monoxide

829. Which of the following toxicant-toxicity pairs is incorrect?

A. aluminum-nystagmus
B. lead–IQ deficits
C. inorganic mercury–tremor
D. manganese–Parkinson's disease

830. All of the following are associated with axonopathies except _____.

A. n-hexane
B. isoniazid
C. nitrofurantoin
D. nicotine

831. Which of the following toxicant-toxic results pairs is incorrect?

A. metronidazole-seizures
B. lithium-ataxia

C. colchicine–blindness

D. dapsone–peripheral neuropathy

832. Which of the following toxicant-association pairs is incorrect?

A. carbon disulfide–waltzing syndrome

B. tri-o-cresyl phosphate–OP-induced delayed neurotoxicity

C. acrylamide–peripheral neuropathy

D. pyridinethione–used in shampoos

833. All of the following are associated with myelinopathies except
_____.

A. amiodarone

B. cisplatin

C. perhexiline

D. tellurium

834. The neurotoxicity of cocaine is mediated by _____.

A. blockade of cholinergic receptors

B. stimulation of muscarinic receptors

C. alteration in striatal dopamine transmission

D. stimulation of NMDA receptors

835. One cause for hepatic encephalopathy is excessive brain levels
of _____.

A. ammonia

B. glucose

C. free fatty acids

D. glutathione

836. A theory for the neurotoxicity of metronidazole is that its
metabolites closely resemble _____.

A. nicain

B. biotin

    C. vitamin B12

    D. thiamine

837. Exposure to fluoroacetate can occur through use of _____.

    A. fluoride toothpaste

    B. Freon

    C. 5-fluorouracil

    D. halothane

838. Nicotine receptors are located in all of the following areas except _____.

    A. ganglia

    B. pancreas

    C. neuromuscular junction

    D. CNS

839. Chinese restaurant syndrome is thought to be due to consumption of excessive amounts of _____.

    A. tyramine

    B. glycine

    C. tyrosine

    D. glutamate

840. MPP+ is transported into the CNS by the same system that transports _____.

    A. glucose

    B. amino acids

    C. dopamine

    D. free fatty acids

841. Peripheral neuropathies from axonopathies are first to involve _____.

    A. midline area of the body

    B. dorsal surface of arms and legs

C. cranial nerves

D. distal parts of hands and feet

842. Which of the following agents promotes the formation of microtubules instead of their depolymerization?

A. vincristine

B. colchicine

C. vinblastine

D. paclitaxel

843. The mechanism of neurotoxicity for hexachlorophene is _____.

A. depletion of CNS dopamine

B. Wallerian degeneration

C. axonopathy

D. intramyelinic edema

844. Which of the following is classified as an amphetamine?

A. MDMA

B. cocaine

C. phenylephrine

D. pseudoephedrine

845. All of the following are true regarding HIV-associated dementia except _____.

A. Cocaine causes a synergistic neurotoxicity.

B. It can be attenuated by beta-estradiol.

C. Amphetamine causes a synergistic neurotoxicity.

D. Cigarette use causes a synergistic neurotoxicity.

846. The main excitatory neurotransmitter of the brain is _____.

A. acetylcholine

B. glycine

C. tryptophan

D. none of the above

847. MPTP is converted to a charged ion by _____.

A. MAO-B
B. MAO-A
C. COMT
D. dopa-decarboxylase

848. Solvent neurotoxicity to the CNS correlates with _____.

A. boiling point
B. vapor pressure
C. lipid solubility, as measured by the air–olive oil partition coefficient
D. none of the above

849. A trigeminal neuropathy could result from chronic exposure to _____.

A. benzene
B. lead
C. dioxin
D. trichloroethylene

850. All of the following are neurologic consequences of carbon monoxide poisoning except _____.

A. carotid artery occlusion
B. Parkinson's disease
C. residual memory deficits
D. MRI abnormalities in subcortical white matter

851. Nitrous oxide can cause neurotoxicity by interfering with _____.

A. vitamin B6
B. vitamin B12
C. folic acid
D. vitamin A

852. Which of the following is least useful in the evaluation of a patient with neurotoxicity?

    A. nerve conduction study
    B. MRI
    C. aspartate transaminase
    D. neuropsychological testing

853. The acute effects of organophosphates are those of _____.

    A. parasympathetic and sympathetic blockade
    B. muscarinic and nicotinic overstimulation
    C. parasympathetic blockade
    D. sympathetic overstimulation

854. All of the following are true regarding exposure to a neurotoxic agent except _____.

    A. They are typically associated with a focal or asymmetric syndrome.
    B. Toxicity is usually dose related.
    C. There is a strong temporal relationship.
    D. A single toxin/toxicant can be associated with multiple neurologic syndromes.

855. A toxicant exposure combined with age-related attrition of neurons is a possible explanation for all of the following except _____.

    A. Parkinson's disease
    B. amyotropic lateral sclerosis
    C. multiple sclerosis
    D. Alzheimer's dementia

856. Statins and ethanol are both associated with _____.

    A. cranial nerve palsy
    B. multiple sclerosis

    C. myopathy

    D. neurotransmitter-associated toxicity

857. Which of the following statements is true regarding polyneuropathies?

    A. Nerve biopsy is always necessary for proper diagnosis.

    B. About 50 % to 66 % of cases remain undiagnosed after medical investigation.

    C. There are no nontoxic causes for polyneuropathy.

    D. Neurologic deficits are often more pronounced in the hands compared to the feet.

858. Which of the following has the highest energy requirement to perform normal functions?

    A. central nervous system neuron

    B. astrocyte

    C. Schwann cell

    D. oligodendrocyte

859. All of the following statements are true except _____.

    A. A single nerve cell can extend to over 1 meter.

    B. The Nissl substance is the site of protein synthesis in neurons.

    C. The central and peripheral nervous systems have equal regenerative abilities.

    D. The blood-brain barrier is incompletely developed at birth.

860. The cell type responsible for the formation of myelin in the central nervous system is the _____.

    A. Schwann cell

    B. oligodendrocyte

    C. glia cell

    D. stellate cell

861. Trimethytin produces a/an _____.

    A. neuronopathy
    B. axonopathy
    C. myelinopathy
    D. blockade of neurotransmitter reuptake

862. The identical axonopathy produced by n-hexane is also produced by _____.

    A. methylmercury
    B. benzene
    C. methyl n-butyl ketone
    D. hexachlorophene

863. Covalent cross-linking of neurofilaments is thought to underlie the nervous system toxicity of _____.

    A. vincristine and vinblastine
    B. amiodarone and tellurium
    C. lead and mercury
    D. carbon disulfide and n-hexane

864. The human neuropathy of lead is unique in that _____.

    A. It is reversible with vitamin B6 intake.
    B. It affects children and not adults.
    C. It presents with predominantly motor symptoms.
    D. There is no clear exposure-response relationship.

865. The cell that appears to be a primary means of defense against toxicant exposure in the CNS is _____.

    A. astrocyte
    B. Schwann cell
    C. oligodendrocyte
    D. Wallerian cell

866. All of the following produce neurotransmission-associated neurotoxicity except _____.

    A. nicotine
    B. metronidazole
    C. cocaine
    D. amphetamine

867. A domoic acid exposure in Canada caused a neurological syndrome because domoic acid is an analog of _____.

    A. glycine
    B. glutamate
    C. GABA
    D. nicotine

868. All of the following are true of excitatory neurotransmitters except _____.

    A. Their toxicity has been implicated in neurodegenerative disease.
    B. Glutamate is the main excitatory neurotransmitter of the brain.
    C. Kainate is 100 times more potent than glutamate.
    D. Benzodiazepines block the excitatory amino acid receptor.

869. A meperidine derivative that is neurotoxic is _____.

    A. GABA
    B. MPTP
    C. GHB
    D. PCP

870. A common toxicologic mechanism for chemicals causing Parkinson's disease is _____.

    A. mitosis arrest
    B. impairment of sodium influx
    C. mitochondrial dysfunction
    D. similarity to endogenous amino acids

871. The neurotoxic metabolite of MPTP _____.

    A. crosses the blood-brain barrier by active transport
    B. is formed in astrocytes by MAO-B
    C. is a free radical
    D. none of the above

872. All of the following are developmental neurotoxicants except _____.

    A. lead
    B. ethanol
    C. folic acid
    D. methylmercury

873. Toxicant-induced amyotrophic lateral sclerosis has been caused by _____.

    A. aluminum
    B. MPTP
    C. paraquat
    D. none of the above

874. Bilirubin and hexachlorophene are most toxic to a/an _____.

    A. premature infant
    B. newborn
    C. immunosuppressed individual
    D. elderly individual

Matching Test

875. amantadine   A. withdrawal seizures

876. clarithromycin   B. myoclonus, hyperreflexia

877. beta-adrenergic blockers C. concentration-related seizure disorder

878. carbon monoxide   D. depression

879. meperidine metabolite E. muscle toxicity

880. lovastatin   F. mania

881. barbiturates   G. psychosis

882. salicylates   H. VIII cranial nerve toxicity

883. *Clostridium* tetani toxin I. Parkinson's disease

CHAPTER 14 ANSWERS (REFERENCES)

818. D (I)
819. C (I)
820. B (I)
821. D (I)
822. A (I)
823. B (I)
824. B (I)
825. D (I)
826. A (I)
827. C (I)
828. A (I)
829. A (I)
830. D (I)
831. C (I)
832. A (I)
833. B (I)
834. C (I)
835. A (I)
836. D (I)
837. C (I)
838. B (I)
839. D (I)
840. C (I)
841. D (I)
842. D (I)
843. D (I)
844. A (I)
845. D (I)
846. D (I)
847. A (I)
848. C (II)
849. D (III)
850. A (III)
851. B (III)
852. C (III)
853. B (III)

854. A (III)
855. C (III)
856. C (III)
857. B (III)
858. A (I)
859. C (I)
860. B (I)
861. A (I)
862. C (I)
863. D (I)
864. C (I)
865. A (I)
866. B (I)
867. B (I)
868. D (I)
869. B (I)
870. C (I)
871. B (I)
872. C (I)
873. D (I)
874. A (I)
875. G (IV)
876. F (IV)
877. D (IV)
878. I (IV)
879. C (IV)
880. E (IV)
881. A (IV)
882. H (IV)
883. B (IV)

REFERENCES

CHAPTER 14

I.   V. C. Moser, M . Aschner, R. J. Richardson, and M. A. Philbert, "Toxic Responses of the Nervous System," in *Casarett & Doull's Toxicology: The Basic Science of Poisons*, 7th ed., ed. C. D. Klaassen (New York: McGraw-Hill, 2008), 631–664.

II. J. Rosenberg and E. A. Katz, "Solvents," in *Current Occupational and Environmental Medicine*, 4th ed., ed. J. Landou (New York: McGraw-Hill, 2007), 481–514.

III. Y. T. So, "Neurotoxicology," in *Current Occupational and Environmental Medicine*, 4th ed., ed. J. Landou (New York: McGraw-Hill, 2007), 373–383.

IV. R. B. Rao, "Neurologic Principles," in *Goldfrank's Toxicologic Emergencies*, 9th ed., ed L. S. Nelson (New York: McGraw-Hill, 2011), 275–284.

15

OCULAR TOXICOLOGY

884. The first site of action for the eye after exposure to a toxicant is the _____.

    A. cornea
    B. tear film
    C. sclera
    D. conjunctiva

885. All of the following statements are true regarding the corneal stroma except _____.

    A. It makes up 90 % of the corneal thickness.
    B. Water-soluble chemicals easily penetrate it.
    C. It can act as a reservoir for toxicants.
    D. It is composed of water, collagen, and glycosaminoglycans.

886. A systemic water-soluble toxicant orally ingested would have the least exposure to the _____.

    A. anterior surface of the lens
    B. corneal endotheliun
    C. aqueous humor
    D. corneal epithelium

887. Electrophysiologic procedures used to test the effects of toxicants on visual function include all of the following except _____.

A. EKG
B. EOG
C. VEP
D. ERG

888. Chemical toxicity is usually associated with what type of color vision deficit?

A. blue-yellow
B. red-green
C. orange-purple
D. brown-gray

889. With respect to surfactant damage to the cornea, which of the following orders of damage are true?

A. anionic > cationic > neutral
B. anionic > neutral > cationic
C. cationic > neutral > anionic
D. cationic > anionic > neutral

890. Organic solvents splashed into the eye should be treated with _____.

A. five milliliters of olive oil irrigation followed by water irrigation
B. irrigation with one drop of dish detergent in one gallon of water
C. 0.01 molar sodium bicarbonate solution irrigation
D. copious water irrigation

891. All of the following are true of the lens except _____.

A. It has a dual blood supply.
B. It grows over the life span of an individual.
C. It is metabolically active and maintains an ionic balance.
D. It is composed of approximately two-thirds water and one-third protein.

892. The mammalian retina is very vulnerable to toxicant-induced damage for all of the following reasons except _____.

    A. a high rate of mitochondrial metabolism
    B. a low choroidal blood flow rate
    C. high turnover of rod and cone outer segments
    D. presence of highly fenestrated choriocapillaries

893. All of the following are true regarding rodent retina except _____.

    A. Its toxicology has relevance for toxicant exposure during the early gestation period in humans.
    B. It is easily accessible.
    C. There is no melanin in the choroid.
    D. Rat rods are similar to those in humans and other primates.

894. Degenerative changes in the optic nerve can result from deficiencies in all of the following except _____.

    A. selenium
    B. zinc
    C. thiamine
    D. B12

895. An antituberculosis drug associated with eye toxicity is _____.

    A. isoniazid
    B. ethambutol
    C. doxycycline
    D. imipenem

896. Solvents that selectively damage the optic nerve and tract are _____.

    A. ethanol and propanol
    B. acetone and chlorobenzene

C. carbon disulfide and acrylamide

D. octane and heptane

897. A chemical used to assess corneal damage is _____.

A. boric acid

B. hypertonic saline

C. indocyanine green

D. fluorescein

898. The slit lamp microscope is least useful in evaluating the _____.

A. retina

B. lens

C. cornea

D. aqueous humor

899. Acute angle closure glaucoma can be precipitated by _____.

A. beta-blockers

B. organophosphate pesticides

C. anticholinergic drugs

D. morphine

900. Inorganic lead exposure has been associated with all of the following except _____.

A. amblyopia

B. glaucoma

C. scotoma

D. optic atrophy

901. The area of the brain associated with vision is _____.

A. occipital lobe

B. frontal lobe

C. temporal lobe

D. pons

902. An area of the central nervous system with a weakened blood-brain barrier is _____.

A. temporal lobe
B. medulla
C. optic disk
D. hypothalamus

903. Intraocular melanin has a high-binding affinity for _____.

A. polycyclic aromatic hydrocarbons
B. toxic heavy metals
C. electrophiles
D. all of the above

904. Which of the following statements is true?

A. Only phase 1 drug metabolizing enzymes are present in the eye.
B. Alterations in visual function may be the initial symptom following chemical exposure.
C. The cornea contains a dual blood supply.
D. all of the above

905. Which of the following statements is true?

A. Arsenic is toxic to the lens.
B. Methanol is toxic to the cornea.
C. Aspartame is toxic to the retina.
D. none of the above

906. The most severe damage to the cornea results from contact with _____.

A. strong acids
B. strong bases

C. organic solvents
D. anionic detergents

907. Cataracts have been associated with all of the following except
_____.

    A. opiate analgesics
    B. corticosteroids
    C. naphthalene
    D. phenothiazines

908. Which of the following drugs are toxic to the retina?

    A. tamoxifen
    B. indomethacin
    C. sildenafil citrate
    D. all of the above

909. Digoxin is toxic to the _____.

    A. cornea
    B. lens
    C. retina
    D. none of the above

910. The eye toxicity of methanol results from _____.

    A. methanol
    B. formaldehyde
    C. formic acid
    D. metabolic acidosis

911. Perchloroethylene eye toxicity has been noted in residents living
close to _____.

    A. gasoline stations
    B. dry cleaners

C. oil refineries

D. autobody repair shops

912. Styrene has been associated with _____.

   A. decreased tear production
   B. cataracts
   C. color vision deficits
   D. nystagmus

CHAPTER 15 ANSWERS (REFERENCES)

884. B (I)
885. B (I)
886. D (I)
887. A (I)
888. A (I)
889. D (I)
890. D (I)
891. A (I)
892. B (I)
893. C (I)
894. A (I)
895. B (I)
896. C (I)
897. D (II)
898. A (II)
899. C (I)
900. B (I)
901. A (I)
902. C (I)
903. D (I)
904. B (I)
905. D (I)
906. B (I)
907. A (I)
908. D (I)
909. C (I)
910. C (I)
911. B (I)
912. C (I)

REFERENCES

CHAPTER 15

I.   D. A. Fox and W. K. Boyes, "Toxic Responses of the Ocular and Visual System," in *Casarett & Doull's Toxicology: The Basic Science of Poisons*, 7th ed., ed. C. D. Klaassen (New York: McGraw-Hill, 2008), 665–698.

II. M. E. Blazka and A. W. Hayes, "Acute Toxicity and Eye Irritancy," in *Principles and Methods of Toxicology*, 5th ed., ed. A. W. Hayes (Boca Raton: Taylor & Francis, 2008), 1131–1178.

16

RESPIRATORY TOXICOLOGY

913. Respiratory tract mucus has all of the following functions except _____.

    A. acid neutralizing
    B. bronchodilation
    C. free radical scavenging
    D. antioxidant

914. All of the following species inhale through the nose and mouth except _____.

    A. mouse
    B. dogs
    C. monkeys
    D. humans

915. Surfactant is produced in _____.

    A. Mucus producing cells
    B. Clara cells
    C. type I alveolar cells
    D. type II alveolar cells

916. All of the following are true of type 1 alveolar cells except _____.

    A. They cover approximately 90 % of the alveolar surface.
    B. They can show preferential damage by toxic agents.

C. They have an attenuated cytoplasm.

D. They are cuboidal in shape.

917. Respiratory tract mucus may be dissolved in a fluid produced by _____.

A. macrophages

B. serous cells

C. type I alveolar cells

D. type II alveolar cells

918. In adult humans, the tidal volume is approximately _____.

A. 200 mL

B. 500 mL

C. 1,000 mL

D. 150 mL

919. Increased lung deposition of particles from polluted air can occur _____.

A. during exercise

B. in emphysema

C. in congestive heart failure

D. in pulmonary edema

920. A toxicant will come in contact with the pulmonary capillary bed before the liver during all of the following routes of administration except _____.

A. inhalation

B. intravenous

C. subcutaneous

D. through a nasal-gastric tube

921. All of the following can decrease the diffusion of gases across the alveolar surface except _____.

   A. pulmonary edema
   B. interstitial fibrosis
   C. collection of inflammatory cells (pneumonia)
   D. pulmonary embolus

922. All of the following statements are true except _____.

   A. Epoxide hydrolase can be found in lung and nasal tissue.
   B. The highest level of P-450 enzymes is found in type 1 alveolar cells.
   C. There are different patterns of induction of xenobiotic-metabolizing enzymes in the lung and liver.
   D. Flavin monooxygenases and prostaglandin synthase are present in lung tissue.

923. The gas that is the least water-soluble and can pass most efficiently through the respiratory tract is _____.

   A. carbon monoxide
   B. ozone
   C. nitrogen dioxide
   D. sulfur dioxide

924. Particles trapped in the nasopharyngeal region are usually of mass-median aerodynamic diameter (MMAD)_____.

   A. > 5 μm
   B. 0.2 to 5μm
   C. 100 nm to 200 nm
   D. < 100 nm

925. All of the following statements are true regarding nanoparticles except _____.

    A. They are defined as particles with a diameter of less than 100 nm.
    B. Nanospheres may be more toxic than nanotubes of the same MMAD.
    C. They have an extremely high surface area relative to their mass.
    D. Technologies that produce decreased emissions of larger particles may produce increased amounts of nanoparticles.

926. A fiber with a length of 200 μm and a diameter of 1 μm will be deposited in the airway mostly by the process of _____.

    A. diffusion
    B. sedimentation
    C. impaction
    D. interception

927. An increase in random motion of a submicrometer particle by Brownian motion of air molecules will increase the deposition of the particle by the process of _____.

    A. diffusion
    B. sedimentation
    C. impaction
    D. interception

928. The deposition of particles in the respiratory tract is increased by _____.

    A. breath holding
    B. exercise
    C. bronchoconstriction
    D. all of the above

929. Lung damage from the production of secondary reaction products such as aldehydes and hydroxyperoxides is characteristic of _____.

A. HCl
B. ammonia
C. ozone
D. lead

930. Free radical-mediated damage to the lung is caused by all of the following except _____.

A. ozone
B. nitrogen dioxide
C. tobacco smoke
D. carbon monoxide

931. Unstable and reactive free radicals and reactive oxygen species produced in the lung by toxicants include all of the following except _____.

A. hydroxyl radical
B. peroxynitrate
C. superoxide
D. sodium radical

932. Which of the following cells is least likely to produce reactive oxygen species in the lung?

A. plasma cell
B. neutrophil
C. monocyte
D. macrophage

933. Bronchoconstriction is produced by all of the following except _____.

A. cigarette smoke
B. an increase in intracellular cGMP

    C. an increase in intracellular cAMP

    D. irritant air pollution

934. In terms of gas exchange in the lung, which of the following pairs of pulmonary pathologies are most similar?

    A. bronchoconstriction and pulmonary fibrosis

    B. pulmonary edema and bronchoconstriction

    C. pulmonary edema and pulmonary fibrosis

    D. pulmonary embolus and pulmonary fibrosis

935. A hypothesis for the etiology of toxicant-induced emphysema is that inflammatory cells increase the burden of _____.

    A. reactive oxygen species

    B. elastases

    C. histamine

    D. nitric oxide

936. In a fibrotic reaction to toxicants, the human lung response most closely resembles _____.

    A. idiopathic pulmonary fibrosis

    B. emphysema

    C. allergic alveolitis

    D. infant respiratory distress syndrome

937. The observed increase in the prevalence of asthma is thought to be related to _____.

    A. increased viability of premature infants

    B. air pollution

    C. increased use of beta-blocking drugs

    D. better reporting methods

938. All of the following are probable human lung carcinogens except
_____.

A. sulfur dioxide
B. arsenic
C. nickel
D. chromium

939. The incidence of nasal carcinoma is increased in all of the
following occupations except _____.

A. nickel refiners
B. chromate workers
C. jewelers
D. mustard gas workers

940. All of the following are found in children exposed to passive
smoke except _____.

A. increase in asthma
B. increase in seizure disorders
C. increase in pneumonia
D. increase in middle ear infections

941. Which of the following toxicant–lung disease pairs is incorrect?

A. aluminum dust–interstitial fibrosis
B. cadmium oxide–emphysema
C. beryllium–interstitial granulomatosis
D. isocyanates–lung cancer

942. Which of the following statements regarding fiber size and
asbestos-related lung disease is incorrect?

A. To cause mesothelioma, fiber diameter must be greater than
2 µm.
B. Lung cancer is associated with fibers larger than 10 µm long.
C. Asbestosis is associated with fibers 2 µm long.
D. Mesothelioma is associated with fibers 5 µm long.

943. The underlying mechanism for pulmonary fibrosis in chronic silicosis involves _____.

A. antigen-antibody complexes
B. bronchospasm
C. pulmonary alveolar macrophages
D. increase in interstitial edema

944. Pulmonary edema is caused by acute exposure to all of the following except _____.

A. ozone
B. asbestos
C. nitrogen dioxide
D. beryllium

945. Reduced glutathione levels in bronchoalveolar lavage fluid may indicate _____.

A. bronchial asthma
B. oxidative stress
C. congestive heart failure
D. enzyme induction

946. Particles that enter the airways of MMAD greater than 10 μm are usually _____.

A. dust from earth's crust
B. smoke particles
C. metal fumes
D. nanoparticles

947. Hypersensitivity pneumonitis is caused by all of the following except _____.

A. *Thermoactinomycetes vulgaris*
B. talc
C. toluene diisocyanate
D. trimellitic anhydride

948. Metals implicated in metal fume fever include all of the following except _____.

   A. gold
   B. zinc
   C. copper
   D. magnesium

949. The symptoms of metal fume fever resemble _____.

   A. acute asthmatic attack
   B. flulike illness
   C. pulmonary edema
   D. emphysema

950. A group of conditions that characterizes the lung's reaction to the chronic deposition of mineral dust into the lung are called _____.

   A. hypersensitivity pneumonitis
   B. bronchospastic disorders
   C. inhalation fevers
   D. pneumoconioses

951. A food that has been implicated in causing bronchiolitis obliterans and obstructive patterns on spirometry in workers is _____.

   A. cinnamon
   B. diacetyl in popcorn flavoring
   C. powdered sugar
   D. nutmeg

952. Pleural plaques are a common marker for exposure to _____.

   A. coal dust
   B. zinc oxide fumes
   C. asbestos
   D. engine dust

953. All of the following are mediators of airway smooth muscle tone except _____.

   A. histamine
   B. aldosterone
   C. leukotriene
   D. nitric oxide

954. Emphysema is defined as _____.

   A. an abnormal enlargement of distal airspaces without obvious fibrosis
   B. an abnormal contraction of distal airspaces with fibrotic walls
   C. fibrotic thickening of alveoli with normal airspace size
   D. an abnormal amount of mucus secretion from the proximal bronchi

955. Lung disease caused by particles is associated with _____.

   A. talc
   B. silica
   C. asbestos
   D. all of the above

956. A blood test that assesses pulmonary function is _____.

   A. arterial blood gas
   B. blood urea nitrogen
   C. tryptase
   D. all of the above

957. Exposure to what gas usually doesn't go further than the nose?

   A. ozone
   B. hydrogen sulfide
   C. sulfur dioxide
   D. nitrogen dioxide

958. Pulmonary toxicity has been associated with all of the following therapeutic agents except _____.

   A. cyclophosphamide
   B. theophylline
   C. bleomycin
   D. carmustine

959. Ammonia, chlorine, and formaldehyde produce upper respiratory tract initiation because _____.

   A. They are highly water-soluble.
   B. They are metabolized by sinus cells to reactive toxicants.
   C. They form droplets that settle in the upper airway.
   D. They have such a noxious odor that the victim holds his breath.

960. Toxicants present in cigarette smoke include all of the following except _____.

   A. naphthalene
   B. free radicals
   C. benzopyrene
   D. phosgene

961. Occupational exposure to all of the following metals has been associated with increased risk of lung cancer except _____.

   A. nickel
   B. cadmium
   C. zinc
   D. beryllium

962. Which of the following is the most water-insoluble gas?

   A. sulfur dioxide
   B. ozone
   C. hydrogen sulfide
   D. nitrogen dioxide

Matching Test

963.	asbestos	A.	bronchiolitis obliterans
964.	cadmium oxide	B.	reaction similar to sarcoidosis
965.	isocyanates	C.	pleural mesothelioma
966.	nickel refining	D.	interstitial fibrosis
967.	aluminum dust	E.	highly water-soluble
968.	oxides of nitrogen	F.	eggshell calcification
969.	beryllium	G.	emphysema, cor pulmonale
970.	polytetrafluoroethylene combustion	H.	nasal cavity squamous cell carcinoma
971.	ammonia	I.	occupational asthma
972.	silicosis	J.	polymer fume fever

CHAPTER 16 ANSWERS (REFERENCES)

913. B (I)
914. A (I)
915. D (I)
916. D (I)
917. B (I)
918. B (I)
919. A (I)
920. D (I)
921. D (I)
922. B (I)
923. A (I)
924. A (I)
925. B (I)
926. D (I)
927. A (I)
928. D (I)
929. C (I)
930. D (I)
931. D (I)
932. A (I)
933. C (I)
934. C (I)
935. B (I)
936. D (I)
937. B (I)
938. A (I)
939. C (I)
940. B (I)
941. D (I)
942. A (I
943. C (I)
944. B (I)
945. B (I)
946. A (II)
947. B (II)
948. A (II)

949. B (II)
950. D (II)
951. B (II)
952. C (II)
953. B (I)
954. A (I)
955. D (I)
956. A (I)
957. C (I)
958. B (I)
959. A (I)
960. D (I)
961. C (I)
962. C (I)
963. C (I)
964. G (I)
965. I (I)
966. H (I)
967. D (I)
968. A (I)
969. B (II)
970. J (II)
971. E (I)
972. F (II)

REFERENCES

CHAPTER 16

I.   H. R. Witschi et al., "Toxic Responses of the Respiratory System," in *Casarett & Doull's Toxicology: The Basic Science of Poisons*, 7th ed., ed. C. D. Klaassen (New York: McGraw-Hill, 2008), 609–630.

II.   J. R. Balmes, "Occupational Lung Diseases," in *Current Occupational and Environmental Medicine*, 4th ed., ed. J. Landou (New York: McGraw-Hill, 2007), 310–333.

17

REPRODUCTIVE TOXICOLOGY

973. Human sexual differentiation begins during geatation week _____.

   A. 2
   B. 3
   C. 7
   D. 10

974. Gonadal differentiation is dependent on signals from which of the following genes?

   A. TES
   B. SRY
   C. AND
   D. CAPUT

975. Fetal testicular androgen production is necessary for the development of all of the following except _____.

   A. testicles
   B. ureter
   C. epididymis
   D. seminal vesicles

976. All of the following are true of cryptorchidism except _____.

   A. It follows a recessive pattern of inheritance.
   B. It occurs in 3 % of full-term male births.

    C. It occurs in 30 % of preterm male births.

    D. It is the most common human birth defect.

977. Which of the following statements is true?

    A. The female reproductive system is more susceptible to endocrine disruption.

    B. Both male and female reproductive systems are equally sensitive to endocrine disruption.

    C. Both male and female reproductive systems are relatively insensitive to endocrine disruption.

    D. The male reproductive system is more susceptible to endocrine disruption.

978. The stages of puberty in boys and girls are determined by using _____.

    A. Müllerian scale

    B. anogenital distance

    C. serum cortisol levels

    D. Tanner stages

979. Which of the following statement is true?

    A. Over the last 40 years, the age of onset of puberty has decreased significantly for boys and girls in most countries in the world.

    B. Over the last 40 years, the age of onset of puberty has decreased for boys only throughout most countries in the world.

    C. Over the last 40 years, the age of onset of puberty has decreased for boys only in the United States.

    D. none of the above

980. Direct exposure to estrogens in personal care and natural products can cause _____.

    A. gynecomastia in boys

    B. arrested adrenarche in girls

C. testicular and ovarian cancer later in life

D. all of the above

981. In the laboratory rat, all of the following are standard landmarks of puberty except _____.

A. anogenital distance

B. male prepubertal separation age

C. age of vaginal opening

D. age of first estrus

982. All of the following are potential endocrine-disrupting chemicals except _____.

A. TCDD

B. acetone

C. methoxychlor

D. vinclozolin

983. All of the following drugs can affect the production of gonadotrophins except _____.

A. hydrochlorothiazide

B. reserpine

C. chlorpromazine

D. monamine oxidase inhibitors

984. Testicular castration will cause _____.

A. decreased serum FSH and LH

B. decreased serum FSH and increased serum LH

C. increased serum FSH and decreased serum LH

D. increased serum FSH and LH

985. All of the following are true of ovarian function except _____.

A. Chemicals that damage oocytes will not lead to reduced fertility.

B. About 400 primary ovarian follicles will produce mature ova during a female's reproductive years.

C. Females are born with about 400,000 follicles in each ovary.

D. At age 30, about 25,000 oocytes remain.

986. All of the following are true of uterine weight in the rat except _____.

   A. It correlates with estrogen exposure.
   B. It increases during proestrus.
   C. It varies throughout the estrus cycle.
   D. It is not measured in most reproductive assays.

987. All of the following male reproductive target sites–toxicant pairs are correct except _____.

   A. CNS–dopamine antagonists
   B. pituitary-zinc
   C. pineal-melatonin
   D. paternal developmental toxicity–cyclophosphamide

988. A chemical that has been shown to inhibit energy metabolism in sperm is _____.

   A. TCE
   B. xylene
   C. epichlorhydrin
   D. styrene

989. A class of drugs that could cause erectile dysfunction is _____.

   A. NSAIDs
   B. drugs affecting autonomic nervous system
   C. phosphodiesterase type 5 inhibitors
   D. angiotensin-converting enzyme inhibitors

990. The most important hormone in the production of milk is _____.

   A. serotonin
   B. oxytocin

C. prolactin

D. norepinephrine

991. In humans, maintenance of the corpus luteum to produce progesterone during pregnancy is dependent on _____.

A. pituitary hormones

B. estrogen

C. prolactin

D. human chorionic gonadotrophin

992. Reducing progesterone levels by 50 % at midpregnancy in the rat will cause _____.

A. increase in ambiguous genitalia

B. significant increase in full litter loss

C. increase in breast cancer in offspring at adulthood

D. no effect on pregnancy outcome

993. According to the testicular dysgenesis syndrome, endocrine-disrupting chemicals during male fetal development could cause decreased Leydig cell function and disturbed Sertoli cell function leading to _____.

A. decreased sperm quality

B. testicular cancer

C. hypospadias

D. all of the above

994. All of the following statements are true except _____.

A. Aminoglutethimide feminizes human males during in utero exposure.

B. Human exposure to endocrine-disrupting chemicals can produce a beneficial effect on one tissue and an adverse effect on another tissue.

C. Testosterone produces a U-shaped dose-response curve for spermatogenesis in the rat.

D. Androgen receptor antagonists can become agonists at high concentrations.

995. Miroestrol is _____.

A. a metabolite of DES
B. a product of a fungus
C. produced by marine invertebrates
D. a phytoestrogen

996. Pulp and paper mill effluents contain a chemical that _____.

A. masculinizes the female mosquito fish
B. binds to the estrogen receptor
C. feminizes the male mosquito fish
D. acts as corticosteroid antagonist

997. The herbicide linuron is _____.

A. an androgen agonist
B. an androgen antagonist
C. an estrogen agonist
D. an estrogen antagonist

998. All of the following are environmental antiandrogens except _____.

A. vinclozolin
B. procymidone
C. p, p1-DDE
D. nandrolone

999. An estrogen receptor agonist present in oral contraceptives that enters aquatic systems from human sewage is _____.

A. estradiol
B. DES

C. ethinyl estradiol

D. pregnenolone

1000. The Endocrine Disruptor Screening and Testing Advisory Committee (EDSTAC) recommends all of the following assays as tier 1 screening tests except _____.

A. multigeneration reproductive study
B. uterotropic assay
C. Hershberger assay
D. pubertal female rat assay

1001. There is strong human evidence for adverse female reproductive or developmental effects for all of the following except _____.

A. carbon monoxide
B. dioxins
C. mercury
D. tobacco smoke

1002. All of the following are considered adverse human pregnancy outcomes except _____.

A. spontaneous abortion
B. postterm delivery
C. low birth weight
D. prematurity

1003. All of the following workplace chemicals have OSHA standards based partially on reproductive effects except _____.

A. methanol
B. lead
C. dibromochloropropane
D. ethylene oxide

1004. Shortened anogenital distance would be expected in male infants born to mothers with high prenatal exposure to _____.

A. tobacco smoke
B. phthalate
C. particulate matter air pollution
D. boron

1005. All of the following medical conditions are associated with decreased male fertility except _____.

A. viral orchitis
B. varicocele
C. hypertension
D. Klinefelter's syndrome

1006. All of the following personal habits have exhibited some evidence for adverse male reproductive outcomes except _____.

A. use of artificial sweeteners
B. frequent hot tub use
C. marijuana use
D. cigarette smoking

1007. Risk factors for adverse female reproductive outcomes include all of the following except _____.

A. HIV treatment
B. viral rhinitis
C. ionizing radiation exposure
D. methotrexate use during pregnancy

1008. All of the following chemicals/drugs can alter the onset of pubertal landmarks in rats except _____.

A. TCDD
B. busulfan
C. methoxychlor
D. erythromycin

1009. A plasticizer that causes delayed puberty in the rat due to Leydig cell inhibition is _____.

A. atrazine
B. ketoconazole
C. dibutyl phthalate
D. aniline

1010. An example of a toxicant that can cause infertility in rats by interfering with testicular blood flow is _____.

A. methylmercury
B. cadmium
C. nickel carbonyl
D. hexavalent chromium

1011. Which of the following chemicals causes testicular toxicity in the rat?

A. m-dinitrobenzene
B. ethylene glycol monomethyl ether
C. methoxyacetic acid
D. all of the above

1012. Which of the following characteristics is least likely to affect transport across the placenta?

A. presence of a chlorine atom
B. protein binding
C. degree of ionization
D. molecular size

1013. The time between fertilization and implantation in humans is approximately _____.

A. 12 hours
B. 1 day
C. 3 days
D. 8 days

1014. It has been suggested that in utero exposure to endocrine-disrupter chemicals could be responsible for all of the following except _____.

   A. decreased sperm counts
   B. sexual dysfunction at age 50
   C. increase in cryptorchid testes
   D. increase in testicular cancer

1015. Examples of endocrine disruptor effects on wildlife include all of the following except _____.

   A. sulfur dioxide effects on rodents
   B. DDT metabolites in birds
   C. PCB effects on fish
   D. environmental estrogen effects on domestic animals

1016. Mechanisms by which xenobiotics alter human development include toxicant binding to all of the following except _____.

   A. estrogen receptor
   B. androgen receptor
   C. acetylcholine receptor
   D. retinoic acid receptor

1017. Adverse estrogenic reproductive effects in domestic animals are produced by feeds contaminated with _____.

   A. solanaceous glycoalkaloids
   B. zearalenone from Fusarium
   C. ergot alkaloids from Claviceps
   D. nitrosoamines

1018. Which of the following is an environmental agonist at the androgen receptor?

   A. 17-beta-trenbolone
   B. o,p 1-DDT

C. vinclozolin
D. methoxychlor

1019. The Hershberger assay detects toxicants with _____ .

A. antiestrogen activity
B. antiandrogen activity
C. mutagenic activity
D. hepatic toxicity

1020. The phthalate syndrome in rats includes all of the following except _____ .

A. causation by flutamide
B. decrease in insulin-like 3 peptide hormone synthesis
C. decrease in testosterone synthesis
D. agenesis of the testicles

CHAPTER 17 ANSWERS (REFERENCES)

973. C (I)
974. B (I)
975. B (I)
976. A (I)
977. D (I)
978. D (I)
979. D (I)
980. A (I)
981. A (I)
982. B (I)
983. A (I)
984. D (I)
985. A ()
986. D (I)
987. B (I)
988. C (I)
989. B (I)
990. C (I)
991. D (I)
992. B (I)
993. C (I)
994. A (I)
995. D (I)
996. A (I)
997. B (I)
998. D (I)
999. C (I)
1000. A (I)
1001. B (II)
1002. B (II)
1003. A (II)
1004. B (III)
1005. C (III)
1006. A (III)
1007. B (II)
1008. D (I)

1009. C (I)
1010. B (I)
1011. D (I)
1012. A (I)
1013. D (I)
1014. B (I)
1015. A (I)
1016. C (I)
1017. B (I)
1018. A (I)
1019. B (I)
1020. A (I).

REFERENCES

CHAPTER 17

I.   P. M. D. Foster and L. E. Gray, "Toxic Responses of the Reproductive System," in *Casarett & Doull's Toxicology: The Basic Science of Poisons*, 7th ed., ed. C. D. Klaassen (New York: McGraw-Hill, 2008),761–806.

II. G. C. Windham and A. M. Osorio, "Female Reproductive Toxicology," in *Current Occupational and Environmental Medicine*, 4th ed., ed. J. Landou (New York: McGraw-Hill, 2007), 384–399.

III. A. M. Osorio and G. C. Windham, "Male Reproductive Toxicology," in *Current Occupational and Environmental Medicine*, 4th ed., ed. J. Landou (New York: McGraw-Hill, 2007), 400–412.

18

ENDOCRINE TOXICOLOGY

1021. Secretory granules are unique to endocrine cells that produce _____.

    A. corticosteroids
    B. sex hormones
    C. peptide hormones
    D. aldosterone

1022. The major inhibitory factor for prolactin release is _____.

    A. dopamine
    B. TRH
    C. FSH
    D. GH

1023. Vasopressin is synthesized primarily in _____.

    A. acidophils of the adenohypophysis
    B. basophils of the adenohypophysis
    C. chromophobes of the adenohypophysis
    D. supraoptic nuclei of the hypothalamus

1024. Lisuride and bromocriptine act as _____.

    A. serotonin agonists
    B. dopamine agonists

    C. cholinergic agonists

    D. dopamine antagonists

1025. The zona glomerulosa of the adrenal gland primarily produces
_____.

    A. sex hormones

    B. aldosterone

    C. glucocorticoids

    D. catecholamines

1026. All of the following are true of the fetal adrenal cortex in
primates except _____.

    A. It produces dehydroepiandrosterone, which is converted to
estrogen by the placenta.

    B. Its tissue could be interpreted as a pathologic lesion in a
histologic specimen from a neonatal primate.

    C. It produces parathyroid hormones.

    D. Following birth, it undergoes a rapid regression with
replacement by cells of the postnatal adrenal cortex.

1027. All of the following are known to induce phospholipidosis
except _____.

    A. phenobarbital

    B. chloroquine

    C. triparanol

    D. chlorphentermine

1028. Cortexolone acts by _____.

    A. inhibiting the synthesis of adrenocorticoids

    B. blocking the release of adrenocorticoids

    C. inhibiting the synthesis of mineralocorticoids

    D. blocking the action of adrenocorticoids at peripheral sites

1029. An assessment of the function of the adrenal cortex is provided by all of the following except _____.

    A. 24-hour urine for cortisol
    B. 24-hour urine for metanephrine
    C. morning serum cortisol
    D. cortisol response to exogenous ACTH

1030. The protein responsible for the transport of iodide into the thyroid follicular lumen is _____.

    A. activin
    B. pendrin
    C. transportin
    D. connexin

1031. Thyroxine is bound to thyroxine-binding globulin in all of the following species except _____.

    A. monkeys
    B. rats
    C. humans
    D. dogs

1032. The cellular mechanism and duration of action of thyroid hormones is similar to _____.

    A. prostaglandins
    B. cytokines
    C. steroid hormones
    D. leukotrienes

1033. Sensitive species for the development of goiters after sulfonamide exposure include all of the following except _____.

    A. rat
    B. mouse
    C. dog
    D. guinea pig

1034. The most common endocrine neoplasm in humans is _____.

    A. pituitary carcinoma
    B. adrenal carcinoma
    C. parathyroid carcinoma
    D. thyroid carcinoma

1035. An increased incidence of thyroid C cell tumors in rats was reported with _____.

    A. a glucagon-like peptide-1 receptor agonist
    B. an ACTH antagonist
    C. a dopamine agonist
    D. an estrogen antagonist

1036. Mutations in the ret proto-oncogene are involved in the hereditary form of _____.

    A. parathyroid carcinoma
    B. adrenal cortex carcinoma
    C. medullar thyroid carcinoma
    D. islet cell carcinoma of the pancreas

1037. Five percent of extracellular calcium is complexed to all of the following except _____.

    A. chloride ion
    B. citrate ion
    C. phosphate ion
    D. bicarbonate ion

1038. A drug that causes an increased incidence of ovarian tumors in mice in a 2-year study is _____.

    A. imipenem
    B. doxycycline
    C. clindamycin
    D. nitrofurantoin

1039. All of the following would lead to increased ovarian tumorigenesis in mice except _____.

    A. exogenous estrogen administration
    B. cytotoxic drugs or radiation
    C. genetic absence of ovarian follicles
    D. autoimmune destruction of oocyte

1040. Experimental diabetes mellitus in animals can be produced by destroying beta cells with _____.

    A. chloramphenicol
    B. streptozocin
    C. phenylbutazone
    D. phenyramidol

1041. All of the following drugs have been associated with acute pancreatitis except _____.

    A. propanolol
    B. azathioprine
    C. thiazides
    D. lisinopril

1042. Hormones secreted from the islets of Langerhans in the pancreas include all of the following except _____.

    A. insulin
    B. somatostatin
    C. gastrin
    D. glucagon

1043. All of the following inhibit adrenocortical steroid biosynthesis except _____.

    A. metyrapone
    B. lithium
    C. aminoglutethimide
    D. mitotane (o' p'-DDD)

1044. Tests that assess the metabolic effects of thyroid hormone include all of the following except _____.

A. systolic time intervals
B. aspartate transaminase
C. basal metabolic rate
D. serum cholesterol

1045. Actions of vasopressin include all of the following except _____.

A. vasoconstriction
B. calcium excretion
C. free water reabsorption
D. corticotropin secretion

1046. All of the following are associated with oxytocin except _____.

A. enhanced sexual arousal in males
B. increased tolerance to pain
C. reduced anxiety
D. uterine relaxation in late labor

1047. All of the following will increase growth hormone levels except _____.

A. arginine
B. L-DOPA
C. somatostatin
D. clonidine

1048. Which of the following hormone-effect pairs is incorrect?

A. ACTH–secretion of glucocorticoids
B. prolactin–synthesis of melanin
C. TSH–secretion of thyroid hormone
D. growth hormone–promotes growth

1049. Which of the following hormone–chemical class pairs is incorrect?

A. prostaglandins–fatty acids
B. insulin-protein
C. TRH–biogenic amine
D. estrogen-steroid

1050. All of the following are true regarding calcium in the human body except _____.

A. The cytosolic calcium concentration is 10,000 times higher than the extracellular fluid concentration.
B. Ninety-nine percent of body calcium is present in bone.
C. Free calcium in serum will increase in the presence of acidosis.
D. Protein-bound calcium is predominantly on albumin.

1051. Which of the following will affect the parathyroid glands the least?

A. ozone
B. aluminum
C. L-asparaginase
D. sulfur dioxide

1052. A drug/chemical that appears to cause an increased incidence of parathyroid adenomas in rats is _____.

A. amiodarone
B. minocycline
C. nicardipine
D. rotenone

1053. Recombinant human parathyroid hormone _____.

A. is a treatment for hypercalcemia
B. is associated with osteosarcoma in rats
C. is a treatment for Paget's disease
D. is associated with hypertension in humans

1054. All of the following are true of parathyroid hormone–related protein except _____.

A. It is present in human tumors.
B. It plays a role in calcium balance in the fetus.
C. It has no structural similarity to parathyroid hormone.
D. It is found in high concentrations in milk.

1055. A contaminant of drinking water from combustible products that can inhibit the transport of iodide into the thyroid is _____.

A. sulfuric acid
B. lead
C. perchlorate
D. none of the above

1056. Chemicals/drugs that inhibit the organification of thyroglobulin include all of the following except _____.

A. thiourea
B. sulfonamides
C. methimazole
D. furosemide

1057. A xenobiotic that inhibits thyroid hormone release is _____.

A. atrazine
B. lithium
C. DDT
D. arsenic

1058. Which of the following statements is not correct?

A. Phenobarbital treatment in rats can increase serum TSH by inducing glucuronidation enzymes.
B. Phenobarbital is a thyroid gland tumor promoter in some animal studies.

C. Epileptic patients on phenobarbital do not have an increased risk of thyroid neoplasms.

D. Epileptic patients on phenobarbital have an increased risk of liver neoplasms.

1059. Mechanisms of toxicity to the adrenal cortex include all of the following except _____.

A. activation of the fetal adrenal gene
B. impaired steroidogenesis
C. toxin activation by P450 enzymes
D. lipidosis-producing chemicals

1060. Captopril is _____.

A. an inhibitor of cholesterol ACYL transference
B. an inhibitor of 21-alpha hydroxylase
C. an inhibitor of tyrosine hydroxylase
D. an inhibitor of angiotensin converting enzyme

1061. Adrenal medullary proliferation tumors are called _____.

A. adrenal adenomas
B. pheochromocytomas
C. mesotheliomas
D. none of the above

1062. A xenobiotic associated with causing pituitary tumors in humans is _____.

A. phenobarbital
B. bromocriptine
C. cobalt
D. none of the above

1063. The active transport of iodide anion can be inhibited by _____.

A. thiocyanate
B. bicarbonate

C. lactate
D. acetate

1064. A food additive that causes inhibition of 5^1-monodeiodinase in the rat is _____.

A. red dye # 3
B. orange B
C. yellow # 5
D. blue # 1

1065. Papillary thyroid carcinoma in humans is strongly related to _____.

A. polio virus
B. rifampin
C. radiation exposure
D. TCDD

1066. The observed gender differences in thyroid cancer prevalence in humans suggest that _____.

A. Androgens play a role in tumorigenesis.
B. Estrogens play a role in tumorigenesis.
C. Body weight plays a role in tumorigenesis.
D. Age plays a role in tumorigenesis.

1067. Thyroid C cells are known to have receptors for hormones produced in _____.

A. adrenal medulla
B. central nervous system
C. gastrointestinal tract
D. kidney

1068. Calcium concentration in body fluids is regulated by all of the following except _____.

A. calcitonin

B. vitamin D
C. parathyroid hormone
D. angiotensin II

1069. The most common endocrine organ to be affected by chemicals is _____.

A. pancreas
B. parathyroid gland
C. adrenal gland
D. pituitary gland

1070. Pituitary tumors in rats are caused by _____.

A. hydocortisone
B. calcitonin
C. angiotensin II
D. none of the above

1071. Which of the following is true regarding Leydig cell tumors?

A. They are the most common testicular neoplasm in humans.
B. They are caused by xenobiotics with androgen agonist activity.
C. Ninety percent of human tumors are malignant.
D. The rat is an inappropriate model for assessing risk of xenobiotic-induced tumor in humans.

1072. All of the following are true of raloxifene except _____.

A. It is associated with increased risk of ovarian cancer in women.
B. It is an estrogen agonist on bone and estrogen antagonist on breast.
C. It increases circulating LH levels in mice.
D. It is associated with ovarian tumor development in mice.

CHAPTER 18 ANSWERS (REFERENCES)

1021.	C (I)	1057.	B (I)
1022.	A (I)	1058.	D (I)
1023.	D (I)	1059.	A (I)
1024.	B (I)	1060.	D (I)
1025.	B (I)	1061.	B (I)
1026.	C (I)	1062.	D (I)
1027.	A (I)	1063.	A (I)
1028.	D (I)	1064.	A (I)
1029.	B (I)	1065.	C (I)
1030.	B (I)	1066.	B (I)
1031.	B (I)	1067.	C (I)
1032.	C (I)	1068.	D (I)
1033.	D (I)	1069.	C (I)
1034.	D (I)	1070.	B (I)
1035.	A (I)	1071.	D (I)
1036.	C (I)	1072.	A (I)
1037.	A (I)		
1038.	D (I)		
1039.	A (I)		
1040.	B (II)		
1041.	A (II)		
1042.	C (II)		
1043.	B (II)		
1044.	B (II)		
1045.	B (II)		
1046.	D (II)		
1047.	C (II)		
1048.	B (II)		
1049.	C (II)		
1050.	A (I)		
1051.	D (I)		
1052.	D (I)		
1053.	B (I)		
1054.	C (I)		
1055.	C (I)		
1056.	D (I)		

REFERENCES

CHAPTER 18

I.   C. C. Capen, "Toxic Responses of the Endocrine System," in *Casarett & Doull's Toxicology: The Basic Science of Poisons*, 7th ed., ed. C. D. Klaassen (New York: McGraw-Hill, 2008), 807–880.

II. R. W. Kapp and J. A. Thomas, "Hormone Assays and Endocrine Function," in *Principles and Methods of Toxicology*, 5th ed., ed. A. W. Hayes (Boca Raton: CRC Press, 2008), 1713–1754.

19

METAL TOXICOLOGY

1073. A property of metals of great toxicologic significance is
_____.

A. They all exhibit a U-shaped dose-response curve.
B. They have no threshold for toxicity.
C. They are less toxic as cations.
D. They accumulate in the biosphere.

1074. A chemical property of elemental metals that makes them
particularly troubling to biological systems is _____.

A. They are essentially nonbiodegradable.
B. They mostly convert to cations with +1 charge.
C. They form insoluble salts.
D. They form alloys.

1075. All of the following are chemical ways that metals cause
toxicity except _____.

A. binding to sulfhydryl groups
B. mimicry of essential metals
C. acting as semiconductors and short-circuiting nerve
impulses
D. acting as catalytic centers for redox reactors in the
generation of reactive oxygen species

1076. One drawback in using hair samples as a tissue to measure metal exposure is that _____.

    A. Metals can be removed from hair by shampoo.
    B. Hair can be contaminated by external sources of metals.
    C. Workers who spend most of their day outside in cold weather will have less hair metal deposition compared to office workers.
    D. Older, graying hair has less reliable deposition rates than younger hair.

1077. Many human metabolites of arsenic are _____.

    A. methylated
    B. sulfated
    C. glucuronidated
    D. acetylated

1078. A recent source of human cadmium exposure is _____.

    A. batteries
    B. synthetic motor oil
    C. dental fillings
    D. crack cocaine

1079. The metal salt of lowest toxicological significance is _____.

    A. vanadium pentoxide
    B. titanium dioxide
    C. thallium sulfate
    D. uranyl chloride

1080. In occupationally exposed adult workers, OSHA standards require the maintenance of blood lead levels below _____.

    A. 10 µg/dL
    B. 20 µg/dL
    C. 40 µg/dL
    D. 80 µg/dL

1081. All of the following may result from lead toxicity to the kidney except _____.

   A. hypouricemia
   B. aminoaciduria
   C. glycosuria
   D. phosphaturia

1082. Which of the following is least useful in a medical evaluation of a lead-exposed worker?

   A. blood pressure measurement
   B. blood lead level
   C. serum creatine phosphokinase (CPK)
   D. microscopic urinalysis

1083. Alcohol intake may influence metal toxicity by all of the following except_____.

   A. altering diet
   B. induction of CYP450 2E1
   C. reduction of essential mineral intake
   D. altering hepatic iron deposition

1084. All of the following are adaptive responses to metal toxicity except _____.

   A. increased albumin synthesis
   B. lead-inclusion bodies
   C. overexpression of metallothionein
   D. metal-induced oxidative stress response

1085. Which of the following metal–medicinal use pairs is incorrect?

   A. platinum–cancer chemotherapy
   B. gold-arthritis
   C. aluminum-dementia
   D. lithium-mania

1086. Enviromental arsenic exposure occurs mainly through _____.

    A. industrial air pollution
    B. automobile exhaust
    C. cigarette smoke
    D. drinking water

1087. A gas with a similar toxicologic effect to arsine is _____.

    A. chlorine
    B. ethane
    C. stibine
    D. ammonia

1088. The combination of nickel with carbon monoxide produces the respiratory tract toxicant _____.

    A. nickel carbonate
    B. phosgene
    C. stilbene
    D. nickel carbonyl

1089. Fluorosis refers to symptoms secondary to excess fluoride intake in _____.

    A. liver and kidney
    B. heart and skeletal muscle
    C. teeth and bones
    D. central and peripheral nervous system

1090. Acrodynia is a disease in children caused by exposure to _____.

    A. arsenic
    B. lead
    C. cadmium
    D. mercury

1091. Mercury is deposited in bodies of water and the atmosphere
_____.

A. through volcanic emissions
B. through industrial emissions
C. through rainwater
D. all of the above

1092. Stainless steel welding exposes workers to all of the following
except _____.

A. chromium
B. sulfur dioxide
C. nickel
D. manganese

1093. Pigmentation of the skin and eyes is associated with prolonged
exposure to _____.

A. silver
B. thallium
C. germanium
D. cesium

1094. Selenium deficiency is associated with _____.

A. seizures
B. peripheral neuropathy
C. cardiomyopathy
D. renal failure

1095. All of the following are associated with beryllium exposure
except _____.

A. lung cancer
B. acute chemical pneumonitis
C. chronic granulomatous disease
D. peptic ulcer disease

1096. All of the following are true regarding mercury exposure except _____.

    A. Sea mammals have higher levels than herbivorous fish do.
    B. Drinking water is a significant source of exposure.
    C. Concentrations in marine life can be 80,000 times higher than in the surrounding water.
    D. Cooking fish does not lower the level of methylmercury.

1097. Which of the following statements is true?

    A. Methylmercury does not cross the placenta.
    B. Methylmercury is metabolized to mercuric ion by the placenta.
    C. Methylmercury is present in the fetal brain at 50 % of the concentration in the maternal blood.
    D. Methylmercury is present in the fetal brain at 5–7 times the concentration in maternal blood.

1098. Which of the following metal–commercial product pairs is incorrect?

    A. zirconium-deodorants
    B. tungsten-detergents
    C. selenium–dandruff shampoos
    D. aluminum-antacids

1099. A metal that substitutes for calcium in bone is _____.

    A. lithium
    B. cesium
    C. silver
    D. strontium

1100. Which of the following is considered a metalloid?

    A. beryllium
    B. bromine

C. boron

D. tungsten

1101. Potassium deficiency can result from all of the following except _____.

A. vomiting
B. renal failure
C. diarrhea
D. diuretic use

1102. All of the following are true regarding exposure of metallic sodium or potassium to air except _____.

A. Superoxides may form.
B. Explosions can occur.
C. Particles embedded in skin or eyes should be irrigated with large amounts of water.
D. Dermal and occular burns can lead to liquification necrosis.

1103. Acute gastrointestinal symptoms with gastrointestinal hemorrhage followed by cardiovascular collapse, renal failure, jaundice, and delayed peripheral neuropathy describes the acute toxicology of _____.

A. mercury
B. lead
C. arsenic
D. cadmium

1104. Colicky abdominal pain, headache, fatigue, encephalopathy are associated with acute exposure to _____.

A. inorganic mercury
B. lead
C. mercury vapor
D. cadmium

1105. All of the following are true of thallium except _____.

    A. Toxicity may result from mimicking sodium ion.
    B. Prussian blue is an antidote.
    C. It is one of the most toxic metals.
    D. Significant exposure can result in dermal, cardiac, or neurological toxicity.

1106. All of the following are true of the toxicity of tin except _____.

    A. An outbreak of toxicity occurred in France during the 1950s.
    B. Inorganic tin compounds are relatively nontoxic.
    C. Organic tin compounds can be very neurotoxic.
    D. Inorganic compounds are better absorbed than organic tin compounds.

1107. All of the following are true of uranium compounds except_____.

    A. Renal toxicity is common.
    B. Acute radiation toxicity is more of a concern than chemical toxicity.
    C. They accumulate in bone.
    D. Urine uranium levels correlate with acute exposure.

1108. All of the following are true of zinc except _____.

    A. It induces metallothionein.
    B. Overdose is more of a problem than deficiency.
    C. It is essential for human growth and development.
    D. Zinc oxide is a cause of "metal fume fever."

1109. Dialysis dementia may be due to excess _____.

    A. potassium
    B. phosphate
    C. aluminum
    D. urea

1110. Bismuth salts are used medically to treat all of the following except _____.

A. diarrhea
B. peptic ulcer
C. H. pylori gastritis
D. inflammatory bowel disease

1111. A metal similar to mercury in that it is liquid at or near room temperature is _____.

A. bromine
B. gallium
C. antimony
D. all of the above

1112. All of the following are manifestations of lithium toxicity except _____.

A. tremor
B. liver necrosis
C. diabetes insipidus
D. renal failure

1113. Hereditary hemochromatosis causes _____.

A. increased intestinal absorption of iron
B. decreased bilary excretion of iron
C. decreased renal excretion of iron
D. increased sensitivity of liver cells to normal levels of iron

1114. There is experimental evidence that iron may play a part in the development of _____.

A. atherosclerosis
B. osteosarcoma
C. adrenal insufficiency
D. hypothyroidism

1115. Metal-induced Parkinson's disease is caused by _____.

    A. magnesium
    B. molybdenum
    C. manganese
    D. selenium

1116. Garlic breath is associated with all of the following except _____.

    A. selenium
    B. cyanide
    C. arsenic
    D. thallium

1117. Trivalent chromium has been used medically to _____.

    A. treat depression
    B. improve sleep
    C. lower blood pressure
    D. decrease insulin resistance

1118. Excess copper ingestion in humans has been associated with _____.

    A. liver necrosis
    B. hypertension
    C. pancreatitis
    D. all of the above

1119. All of the following are true in Wilson's disease except _____.

    A. There is impaired biliary excretion of copper.
    B. Serum ceruloplasmin is elevated.
    C. Serum unbound copper levels are elevated.
    D. There are characteristic corneal findings.

1120. Menkes' disease is characterized by _____.

    A. increased liver copper
    B. copper deficiency in the brain
    C. bronze skin
    D. none of the above

1121. All of the following are true of iron deficiency except _____.

    A. It is the most common nutrient deficiency in the world.
    B. The major presentation in young children is seizure disorder.
    C. It is associated with adverse pregnancy outcomes in adults.
    D. It causes a microcytic anemia.

1122. Symptoms of acute iron overdose include _____.

    A. seizures, polyuria, bradycardia
    B. skin rash, respiratory alkalosis, bleeding
    C. parathesias, muscle weakness, tremors
    D. nausea, abdominal pain, metabolic acidosis

1123. The form of mercury that has the highest gastrointestinal absorption is _____.

    A. elemental
    B. mercurous
    C. mercuric
    D. methylmercury

1124. A major toxicokinetic issue with methylmercury is _____.

    A. enterohepatic recycling
    B. storage in bone
    C. renal failure–induced deceased renal excretion
    D. saturation of P-glycoprotein exporter

1125. The major target organ of inorganic mercury is _____.

    A. brain
    B. peripheral nerve
    C. kidney
    D. adrenal gland

1126. The major tragedy of the Minamata, Japan, methylmercury exposure was _____.

    A. lifetime seizure disorder in exposed adults
    B. developmental disabilities in offspring of exposed pregnant mothers
    C. intellectual deficits in exposed children
    D. high incidence of lymphoma in all exposed groups

1127. Excessive cobalt ingestion in humans has been associated with _____.

    A. congestive heart failure
    B. increase in red blood cells
    C. goiter
    D. all of the above

1128. Lead inhibits the activity of _____.

    A. aspartate transaminase
    B. ferrochelatase
    C. beta-glucuronidase
    D. superoxide dismutase

1129. Lead in blood is mostly _____.

    A. in neutrophils
    B. bound to albumin
    C. in erythrocytes
    D. unbound

1130. Biochemical effects of lead include all of the following except
_____.

    A. inhibition of delta-aminolevulinic acid dehydratase
    B. increase in protophorphin IX in erythrocytes
    C. decrease in urine delta-aminolevulinic acid excretion
    D. chelation of zinc by erythrocytes

1131. The most common adverse reaction to nickel is _____.

    A. contact dermatitis
    B. gout
    C. hypertension
    D. pulmonary edema

1132. All of the following are true of methylmercury except _____.

    A. It is produced by biomethylation reactions in oceans.
    B. It can significantly bioconcentrate.
    C. The major human health risk is neurotoxicity.
    D. It can be destroyed by cooking at 160°F.

1133. All of the following are true of arsenic except _____.

    A. It is strongly positive in the Ames test.
    B. Neurologic symptoms after acute exposure are delayed by 1 to 2 weeks.
    C. It is associated with peripheral vascular disease.
    D. Skin cancers frequently occur on palms of hands and soles of feet.

1134. Beryllium exposure is associated with _____.

    A. hemolytic anemia
    B. alopecia
    C. Parkinson's disease
    D. granulomatous lung disease

1135. All of the following are true of cadmium exposure except
_____.

A. Food is a principal source of exposure.
B. It causes proximal tubular dysfunction.
C. It can be associated with bone deformities.
D. Dialysis is an effective treatment.

1136. The toxicity of hexavalent chromium is thought to result from
_____.

A. binding to the estrogen receptor
B. free radical generation during its conversion to trivalent chromium
C. precipitation in the kidney
D. blockade of sodium channels

1137. Lead and cadmium may both be associated with all of the following except _____.

A. proximal tubular renal dysfunction
B. hypertension
C. pancreatitis in humans
D. osteoporosis

1138. Baldness is associated with _____.

A. thallium
B. gold
C. silver
D. cobalt

1139. All of the following are factors that influence metal toxicity except _____.

A. person's age at exposure
B. valence state of metal
C. blood glucose level
D. concurrent alcohol or smoking

1140. Which of the following has the shortest biological half-life?

A. cadmium in kidney
B. lead in bone
C. lithium in blood
D. gold in synovial tissue

1141. All of the following are correct metal–binding protein pairs _____.

A. transferrin-iron
B. C-reactive protein–lead
C. metallothionein-cadmium
D. metallothionein-zinc

1142. Fingernails and hair are good biomarkers for exposure to _____.

A. arsenic
B. magnesium
C. potassium
D. boron

1143. The triad of symptoms traditionally associated with chronic inhalation of mercury vapor are _____.

A. baldness, skin rash, tremors
B. erethism, diarrhea, weight loss
C. psychosis, hematuria, jaundice
D. tremors, gingivitis, erethism

1144. Peripheral neuropathy is not a common manifestation of toxicity with _____.

A. lead
B. arsenic
C. cadmium
D. cisplatin

Matching Test

1145. Cr^{+3}

A. converts Fe^{+2} to Fe^{+3}

1146. phosphate ion

B. Indian childhood cirrhosis

1147. Zn

C. causes increased erythropoiesis

1148. sulfate ion

D. Hepcidin modulates absorption.

1149. ceruloplasmin

E. mimics potassium

1150. Cd

F. essential for glucose metabolism

1151. Co

G. contact dermatitis and epigenetic carcinogen

1152. Fe

H. arsenate mimics

1153. Mn

I. chromate mimics

1154. Se

J. Deficiency causes acrodermatitis enteropathica.

1155. Ni

K. gout

1156. Li

L. toxicity treated with amiloride

1157. Mo

M. present in thioredoxin

1158. Cs

N. present in pesticides

1159. Cu

O. self-tolerance

CHAPTER 19 ANSWERS (REFERENCES)

1073. D (I)	1109. C (I)	1145. F (I)
1074. A (I)	1110. D (I)	1146. H (I)
1075. C (I)	1111. B (I)	1147. J (I)
1076. B (I)	1112. B (I)	1148. I (I)
1077. A (I)	1113. A (I)	1149. A (I)
1078. A (I)	1114. A (I)	1150. O (I)
1079. B (I)	1115. C (I)	1151. C (I)
1080. C (II)	1116. B (I)	1152. D I)
1081. A (II)	1117. D (I)	1153. N (I)
1082. C (II)	1118. A (I)	1154. M (I)
1083. B (I)	1119. B (I)	1155. G (I)
1084. A (I)	1120. B (I)	1156. L (I)
1085. C (I)	1121. B (I)	1157. K (I)
1086. D (I)	1122. D (I)	1158. E (I)
1087. C (I)	1123. D (I)	1159. B (I)
1088. D (II)	1124. A (I)	
1089. C (I)	1125. C (I)	
1090. D (I)	1126. B (I)	
1091. D (I)	1127. D (I)	
1092. B (II)	1128. B (I)	
1093. A (I)	1129. C (I)	
1094. C (I)	1130. C (I)	
1095. D (I)	1131. A (I)	
1096. B (I)	1132. D (I)	
1097. D (I)	1133. A (I)	
1098. B (III)	1134. D (I)	
1099. D (III)	1135. D (I)	
1100. C (III)	1136. B (I)	
1101. B (III)	1137. C (I)	
1102. C (III)	1138. A (I)	
1103. C (II)	1139. C (I)	
1104. B (II)	1140. C (I)	
1105. A (I)	1141. B (I)	
1106. D (I)	1142. A (I)	
1107. B (I)	1143. D (I)	
1108. B (I)	1144. C (I)	

REFERENCES

CHAPTER 19

I.   J. Liu, R. A. Goyer, and M. P. Waalkes, "Toxic Effects of Metals," in *Casarett & Doull's Toxicology: The Basic Science of Poisons*, 7th ed., ed. C. D. Klaassen (New York: McGraw-Hill, 2008), 931–980.

II.   R. Lewis, "Metals," in *Current Occupational and Environmental Medicine*, 4th ed., J. Landou (New York: McGraw-Hill, 2007), 413–438.

III.   J. C. Merrill, J. J. P. Morton, and S. D. Soleau, "Metals," in *Principles and Methods of Toxicology*, 5th ed., ed. A. W. Hayes (Boca Raton: Taylor and Francis, 2008), 841–896.

20

CHEMICAL AND SOLVENT TOXICOLOGY

1160. All of the following are inducers of P450 2E1 except _____.

    A. acetone
    B. ethanol
    C. isoniazid
    D. phenobarbital

1161. Which of the following can affect the toxicity of solvents?

    A. time of day
    B. diet
    C. physical activity
    D. all of the above

1162. A metabolite of trichloroethylene that is also a metabolite of a marketed sedative for children is _____.

    A. trichloroethylene epoxide
    B. trichloroethanol
    C. trichloromethane
    D. dichlorethylene

1163. The strongest association between high exposure to trichloroethylene and human cancer has been with _____.

    A. malignant melanoma
    B. astrocytoma
    C. renal cell carcinoma
    D. osteosarcoma

1164. An unusual feature of methylene chloride metabolism is _____.

    A. It is auto-inducing.
    B. A metabolite is carbon monoxide.
    C. There are no P450-mediated pathways.
    D. It is metabolized to hydrochloric acid, which causes a metabolic acidosis.

1165. The strongest association between exposure to ethylene glycol monomethyl ether and human disease is _____.

    A. congestive heart failure
    B. infertility in men
    C. biliary stasis
    D. pulmonary fibrosis

1166. Methyl tert-butyl ether _____.

    A. was present in gasoline up to 15 % by volume
    B. causes cancer in animals
    C. is present in groundwater
    D. all of the above

1167. Jet fuels _____.

    A. are predominantly ethers
    B. are toxic to the skin, lung, and immune system in animals
    C. are highly renal toxic in humans
    D. all of the above

1168. All of the following are true of carbon disulfide except _____.

A. It is associated with cognitive impairment.
B. It is a possible risk factor for cardiovascular disease.
C. Elevated carboxyhemoglobin levels are biomarkers of exposure.
D. It is a product of disulfiram metabolism.

1169. All of the following class generalizations for hydrocarbon toxicity are correct except _____.

A. amines/amides-sensitizers
B. aldehydes-irritants
C. decreased lipophilicity–increased CNS depression
D. unsaturated, short chain–animal carcinogens

1170. A unique challenge in evaluating solvent toxicology is that many solvents are _____.

A. flammable
B. mixtures
C. expensive
D. ubiquitous in the environment

1171. All of the following are true in solvent abuse except _____.

A. The blood-brain barrier causes a significant delay between blood levels and brain levels.
B. Almost 20% of eighth graders admit to abusing inhalants.
C. There is a potential for dependence.
D. Death can occur by cardiac arrhythmia.

1172. All of the following statements are true of volatile organic compounds (VOC) except _____.

A. VOCs entering the lung are absorbed into the arterial circulation.
B. VOCs absorbed through the intestine mainly enter the portal circulation.

C. Low doses of many VOCs are metabolized by cytochrome 2D6.
D. The major routes of elimination of VOCs are metabolism and exhalation.

1173. Chronic isopropyl alcohol exposure can potentiate carbon tetrachloride hepatorenal toxicity by _____.

A. additive direct toxic effects
B. induction of metabolism
C. increased absorption
D. decreased first-pass effect

1174. True statements regarding gender differences in solvent disposition include all of the following except _____.

A. Males have more lean body mass.
B. Females have smaller volumes of distribution for polar solvents.
C. Females have higher activity of gastric alcohol dehydrogenase.
D. There are no major differences in P450 metabolism between males and females.

1175. Theories for alcohol-induced hepatotoxicity include all of the following except _____.

A. release of endotoxin
B. binding to the estrogen receptor
C. malnutrition
D. release of inflammatory mediators by Kupffer cells

1176. The site of toxicity for methanol appears to be _____.

A. retinal P450 2E1
B. retinal alcohol dehydrogenase
C. retinal aldehyde dehydrogenase
D. retinal cytochrome c oxidase

1177. The treatment for methanol toxicity can include _____.

   A. dialysis
   B. sodium bicarbonate
   C. methylpyrazole
   D. all of the above

1178. Ethylene glycol causes _____.

   A. acute renal toxicity
   B. peripheral neuropathy
   C. hypercalcemia
   D. all of the above

1179. Propylene glycol _____.

   A. causes reproductive toxicity
   B. is "generally recognized as safe"
   C. is metabolized to oxalic acid
   D. has a major metabolite whose formation cannot be inhibited
      by ethanol

1180. Metabolites of toluene include all of the following except
   _____.

   A. hippuric acid
   B. phenol
   C. benzoic acid
   D. benzyl alcohol

1181. The primary toxic target organ for toluene is _____.

   A. liver
   B. lung
   C. CNS
   D. adrenal gland

1182. Xylene is _____.

    A. present in gasoline
    B. primarily CNS toxic
    C. not genotoxic
    D. all of the above

1183. Styrene _____.

    A. is a solid at room temperature
    B. is chemically divinyl benzene
    C. a definite human respiratory tract carcinogen
    D. none of the above

1184. Populations with a low level of acetaldehyde dehydrogenase would be expected to have _____.

    A. increased risk of alcoholism
    B. increased risk of cancer
    C. increased risk of offspring with fetal alcohol syndrome
    D. none of the above

1185. The highly toxic P450-mediated metabolite of carbon tetrachloride is _____.

    A. hydroxyl radical
    B. chloride radical
    C. chloroform
    D. trichloromethyl radical

1186. The use of carbon tetrachloride has significantly declined because of all of the following issues except _____.

    A. flammability
    B. hepatorenal toxicity
    C. carcinogenicity
    D. ozone depletion

1187. The toxic metabolite of chloroform is thought to be _____.

A. trichloromethyl radical
B. phosgene
C. hypochlorous acid
D. all of the above

1188. All of the following are true of benzene metabolism except _____.

A. Mycloperoxidase may play an important role in bone marrow toxicity.
B. The formation of benzene epoxide is catalyzed by P450 2E1.
C. A metabolite that appears in urine is t, t-muconic acid
D. Quinone oxidoreductase is a liver enzyme that converts benzene to a mylotoxic metabolite.

1189. Benzene exposure has been associated with an increased risk of _____.

A. liver cancer
B. renal cell carcinoma
C. acute myelogenous leukemia
D. lung cancer

1190. All of the following are true of the CNS pharmacology of solvent abuse except _____.

A. It may be similar to alcohol.
B. It has the potential for tolerance.
C. Naloxone will precipitate life-threatening withdrawal reactions.
D. It may involve GABA, glycine, and NMDA receptors.

1191. Which of the following is false?

A. CYP2E1 activity decreases by 80% between the ages of 21 and 65.
B. Polar solvents will reach higher levels in the elderly.

C. Extracellular water is highest in newborns.
D. CYP2E1 is low in fetal liver.

1192. All of the following are true except?

   A. Exercise increases alveolar ventilation rate and cardiac output.
   B. Pulmonary blood flow and pulmonary metabolism are rate limiting for uptake of lipid soluble solvents.
   C. Exercise can increase uptake of both polar and lipid soluble solvents.
   D. Blood flow to liver and kidney increases with exercise.

1193. All of the following are true of trichloroethylene except _____.

   A. DCVC is a reactive metabolite mediated by GSH.
   B. It can stimulate the PPAR alpha-receptor.
   C. It can stimulate the estrogen receptor.
   D. TCAA is a reactive metabolite mediated by CYP P450.

1194. Which of the following is a cyclic ether?

   A. dioxane
   B. dioxin
   C. styrene
   D. A and B

1195. All of the following are true of turpentine except _____.

   A. It is associated with scleroderma.
   B. It is a mixture.
   C. In the same chemical class is d-limonene.
   D. It is associated with allergic contact dermatitis.

1196. Dimethylformamide _____.

   A. is water insoluble
   B. can cause pancreatitis

C. is a solid at room temperature
D. is used by dry cleaners

1197. Evaporation rate _____.

A. is inversely related to lipid solubility
B. is directly related to boiling point
C. is a number without units
D. is another name for vapor pressure

1198. Percutaneous absorption of xylene and toluene vapors in humans _____.

A. is usually insignificant
B. can lead to metabolism in the stratum corneum and production of metabolites that can cause squamous cell carcinoma
C. accounts for about 10 % of total body absorption
D. can be equal to pulmonary absorption in a person who is sweating

1199. Angina pectoris and sudden cardiac death have occurred in _____.

A. painters
B. rayon workers
C. miners
D. dynamite workers

1200. Nitrosamines are formed _____.

A. from a primary amine and hydroxyl ion
B. from a secondary amine and nitrite in an acid medium
C. from a tertiary amine and nitrite in an alkaline medium
D. from a secondary amine and nitrite in an alkaline medium

1201. All of the following are true of styrene except _____.

A. It is a flame retardant.
B. It has an epoxide as a metabolite.

C. It causes neuropsychological deficits in humans.

D. Mandelic acid in urine is a marker of exposure in humans.

1202. Vinyl chloride is associated with _____.

A. proximal tubular necrosis
B. thyroid dysfunction
C. Raynaud's phenomenon
D. peripheral neuropathy

1203. Phenol _____.

A. is highly water-insoluble
B. is well absorbed through the skin
C. is associated with acute leukemia
D. has a half-life of 5 days in humans

1204. Hypocalcemia and hypomagnesemia have occurred in humans after exposure to _____.

A. hydrofluoric acid
B. boric acid
C. tannic acid
D. bromine

1205. Hydrofluoroic acid exposure has been associated with _____.

A. osteosarcoma
B. osteosclerosis
C. hepatitis
D. anemia

1206. Acrylamide exposure has been associated with all of the following except _____.

A. peripheral neuropathy
B. sweating
C. ataxia
D. hypertension

1207. Urinary p-aminophenol is a biologic monitor for exposure to
_____.

A. benzene
B. toluene
C. aniline
D. xylene

1208. All of the following are true of carbon disulfide exposure
except _____.

A. Exposed workers are at an increased risk for cardiovascular
death.
B. Atypical Parkinson's disease has occurred.
C. The eye and ear are target organs.
D. Fifty percent is excreted unchanged by the kidney.

1209. There is debate as to whether or not low exposure to any solvent
could produce _____.

A. carcinogencity
B. liver disease
C. renal disease
D. neuropsychological dysfunction

1210. All of the following are true of volatile organic compounds
(VOCs) except _____.

A. Contamination of drinking water is not a major concern.
B. Atmospheric concentrations are usually low.
C. VOCs in surface water rise to the surface or sink to the bottom.
D. Winds can dilute and disperse solvent vapors to large
distances.

1211. Hypokalemia and normal anion gap metabolic acidosis are
most commonly associated with _____.

A. methyl alcohol
B. octane

C. toluene

D. n-hexane

1212. The most common cause of death in solvent abusers is _____.

A. liver failure
B. renal failure
C. acute lung injury
D. sudden cardiac death

1213. Of the following, the solvent least likely to be abused is _____.

A. ethylene glycol
B. xylene
C. toluene
D. perchloroethylene

1214. Toluene _____.

A. is ethylbenzene
B. causes cholestasis
C. is myelotoxic
D. none of the above

1215. 1,3 butadiene

A. is implicated in cancer in humans
B. can deplete the ozone layer
C. is less reactive than butane
D. all of the above

1216. Which of the following statements is false regarding cyclohexane?

A. It is used in the synthesis of nylon.
B. It is the only cyclic aliphatic hydrocarbon extensively used as an industrial solvent.

C. It causes a peripheral neuropathy similar to n-hexane.

D. It can cause neurobehavioral dysfunction.

1217. The risk of peripheral neuropathy is highest with _____.

A. aromatic petroleum naphtha

B. petroleum ether

C. mineral spirits

D. kerosene

1218. Hepatic angiosarcoma has been associated with all of the following exposures except _____.

A. thorium dioxide

B. naphthalene

C. vinyl chloride

D. arsenic

1219. The most frequently found volatile organ compound (VOC) in finished drinking water supplies in the United States is _____.

A. chloroform

B. carbon tetrachloride

C. 1, 3 butadiene

D. methylene chloride

1220. All of the following are true of organic solvents except _____.

A. Solvents are highly absorbed from the GI tract.

B. Hydrophilic solvents absorbed through inhalation take longer to reach steady state than hydrophobic solvents do.

C. Dermal absorption in rodents is less than in humans.

D. Corn oil can delay the GI absorption of carbon tetrachloride in the rat.

1221. All of the following are possible mechanisms of ethanol carcino-genicity except _____.

   A. Congeners can influence carcinogenicity.
   B. Immune function can be stimulated.
   C. Nutrients can be reduced.
   D. CYP2E1 induction

1222. Known human carcinogens present in gasoline are _____.

   A. benzene and 1, 3 butadiene
   B. hexane and pentane
   C. toluene and xylene
   D. all of the above

1223. Carbon disulfide exposure _____.

   A. may accelerate atherosclerosis
   B. can cause peripheral neuropathy
   C. has been associated with increased blood pressure in workers
   D. all of the above

Matching Test

1224. toluene

A.   low odor threshold

1225. benzidine

B.   inorganic lung carcinogen

1226. acrylonitrile

C.   mist associated with laryngeal cancer

1227. calcium oxide

D.   liver and pancreatic toxicity

1228. chromic acid

E.   depletes ozone in atmosphere

1229. esters

F.   potentiates absorption of other chemicals through the skin

1230. chlorofluorocarbons

G.   azo dyes

1231. dimethyl sulfoxide

H.   may release HCN while burning

1232. dimethylformamide

I.   glue sniffing

1233. sulfuric acid

J.   caustic alkali

CHAPTER 20 ANSWERS (REFERENCES)

1160. D (I)	1196. B (III)	1232. D (III)
1161. D (I)	1197. C (IV)	1233. C (II)
1162. B (I)	1198. A (IV)	
1163. C (I)	1199. D (II)	
1164. B (I)	1200. B (II)	
1165. B (I)	1201. A (II)	
1166. D (I)	1202. C (II)	
1167. B (I)	1203. B (II)	
1168. C (I)	1204. A (II)	
1169. C (I)	1205. B (II)	
1170. B (I)	1206. D (II)	
1171. A (I)	1207. C (II)	
1172. C (I)	1208. D (II)	
1173. B (I)	1209. D (I)	
1174. C (I)	1210. A (I)	
1175. B (I)	1211. C (III)	
1176. D (I)	1212. D (III)	
1177. D (I)	1213. A (III)	
1178. A (I)	1214. D (III)	
1179. B (I)	1215. A (V)	
1180. B (I)	1216. C (III)	
1181. C (I)	1217. B (III)	
1182. D (I)	1218. B (V)	
1183. D (I,II)	1219. A (I)	
1184. B (I)	1220. C (I)	
1185. D (I)	1221. B (I)	
1186. A (I)	1222. A (I)	
1187. B (I)	1223. D (I)	
1188. D (I)	1224. I (III)	
1189. C (I)	1225. G (II)	
1190. C (I)	1226. H (II)	
1191. A (I)	1227. J (II)	
1192. D (I)	1228. B (II)	
1193. C (I)	1229. A (III)	
1194. D (II,III)	1230. E (III)	
1195. A (III)	1231. F (III)	

REFERENCES

CHAPTER 20

I. J. V. Bruckner, S. Satheesh, and D. A. Warren, "Toxic Effects of Solvents and Vapors," in *Casarett & Doull's Toxicology: The Basic Science of Poisons*, 7th ed., ed. C. D. Klaassen (New York: McGraw-Hill, 2008), 981–1052.

II. R. J. Harrison, "Chemicals," in *Current Occupational and Environmental Medicine*, 4th ed., ed. J. Landou (New York: McGraw-Hill, 2007), 439–480.

III. J. Rosenberg and E. A. Katz, "Solvents," in *Current Occupational and Environmental Medicine*, 4th ed., J. Landou (New York: McGraw-Hill, 2007), 481–514.

IV. D. L. Dahlstrom and M. Buckalew, "Solvents and Industrial Hygiene," in *Principles and Methods of Toxicology*, 5ht ed., ed A.W. Hayes (Boca Raton: Taylor and Francis, 2008), 693–726.

V. H. S. Rugo, "Occupational Cancer," in *Current Occupational and Environmental Medicine*, 4th ed., ed. J. Landou (New York: McGraw-Hill, 2007), 224–261.

21

PESTICIDES

1234. An adjunct in the treatment of organophorus poisoning is _____.

A. morphine
B. aminophylline
C. prochlorperazine
D. none of the above

1235. Human male reproductive effects have been demonstrated after exposure to _____.

A. permethrin
B. chlordecone
C. piperonyl butoxide
D. none of the above

1236. Which of the following is the most commonly used rodenticide?

A. strychnine
B. alpha-naphthylthiourea
C. rotenone
D. anticoagulants

1237. Which of the following is a plant growth regulator?

A. gibberellic acid
B. glyphosate

C. simazine

D. asulam

1238. Many of the organochlorine insecticides are no longer in use because of _____.

A. environmental persistence

B. bioaccumulation

C. cancer in laboratory animals

D. all of the above

1239. Piperonyl butoxide _____.

A. is synergistic with pyrethrins

B. has additive activity to pyrethrins because of intrinsic insecticidal activity

C. is a renal toxicant

D. In lab animals, initial induction of P450 is followed by inhibition.

1240. Which of the following has caused thyroid carcinoma in lab animals?

A. warfarin

B. zineb

C. chlordecone

D. dieldrin

1241. The cause of death in acute organophosphate poisoning is usually _____.

A. respiratory failure

B. cardiac arrhythmia

C. status epilepticus

D. hypothermia

1242. All of the following are true of individuals with a genetic predisposition for an abnormal plasma cholinesterase except _____.

A. They have prolonged paralysis after succinylcholine.
B. They have a normal response to curare.
C. They are more susceptible to organophosphates.
D. Dibucaine number is a measure of activity.

1243. The least toxic agent in terms of oral LD50 is _____.

A. parathion
B. alpha-naphthylthiourea (ANTU)
C. aldicarb
D. resmethrin

1244. There have been conflicting studies about the relationships between DDE serum levels and _____.

A. breast cancer
B. osteosarcoma
C. dementia
D. acute leukemia

1245. All of the following organochlorine pesticides are still in use in the United States except _____.

A. dicofol
B. chlordecone
C. endosulfan
D. lindane

1246. The advantage of 2-PAM over atropine in the treatment of organophosphate poisoning is _____.

A. It is helpful in arrhythmias.
B. It suppresses seizures.
C. It acts at the neuromuscular junction.
D. It prevents delayed neuropathy.

1247. Poisoning with chlordecone has been treated with _____.

    A. cholestyramine
    B. propranolol
    C. 2-PAM
    D. none of the above

1248. The mechanism of action of sodium fluoroacetate is _____.

    A. inhibition of glucose-6-phosphate dehydrogenase
    B. inhibition of cytochrome oxidase
    C. inhibition of aconitase
    D. inhibition of DNA polymerase

1249. The acute toxicity of which of the following compounds has been proposed to be due to the presence of surfactant in their formulations? _____.

    A. captan and folpat
    B. glyphosate and glufosinate
    C. atrazine and simazine
    D. alachlor and metolachlor

1250. The primary toxicity of elemental sulfur exposure in humans is _____.

    A. dermatitis
    B. skin cancer
    C. immune suppression
    D. polycythemia

1251. All of the following are true of DDT except _____.

    A. Convulsions can occur in severe poisoning.
    B. The liver is a target organ.
    C. An early symptom of exposure in humans in hyperesthesia of the mouth.
    D. It is a cyclohexane derivative.

1252. The presence of dimethylphosphate in urine is an indication of exposure to _____.

    A. propoxur
    B. dichlorvos
    C. fenvalerate
    D. heptachlor

1253. Paraquat _____.

    A. is a rodenticide
    B. interferes with calcium channels
    C. is well absorbed orally
    D. is transported into the lung

1254. Which of the following is true of diquat?

    A. It is bone marrow toxic.
    B. It causes cataracts in animals.
    C. It is teratogenic.
    D. It accumulates in the liver.

1255. 2, 4, D _____.

    A. is called Agent Orange
    B. is chemically similar to auxin
    C. has been found to contain up to 70 % TCDD
    D. is a chloroacetanilide herbicide

1256. DEET _____.

    A. is cardiotoxic
    B. inhibits photosynthesis
    C. is widely used and has a good safety record
    D. has a high incidence of dermatitis

1257. All of the following are true of imidocloprid except _____.

    A. It is structurally similar to nicotine.
    B. It has selective toxicity for insects over mammals.
    C. It can be toxic to birds.
    D. It has been banned worldwide.

1258. Lepidopteran is an example of a _____.

    A. preemergent herbicide
    B. pheromone
    C. recently introduced pesticide
    D. banned fungicide

1259. A mechanism of action for organotin fungicides is _____.

    A. stimulation of apoptosis
    B. inhibition of succinate dehydrogenase
    C. binding to cytochrome b1
    D. binding to ATP synthase

1260. The toxin from Bacillus thuringiensis is called _____.

    A. delta-endotoxin
    B. bufotalin
    C. batrachotoxin
    D. ciguatoxin

1261. The mechanism of action of triazine herbicides is _____.

    A. activation of auxin receptor
    B. inhibition of photosynthetic electron transport
    C. inhibition of fatty acid synthesis
    D. inhibition of microtubule assembly

1262. Which of the following is true of an uncoupler of mitochondrial respiration?

A. increase in pH of cytoplasm
B. Carboxyhemoglobin increases in red cells.
C. Oxygen consumption increases and ATP production decreases.
D. none of the above

1263. All of the following are symptoms of organophosphorus insecticide poisoning except _____.

A. muscle twitching
B. diarrhea
C. mydriasis
D. vomiting

1264. Oxine therapy 24 hours after exposure to methoxychlor is useless because _____.

A. of the process of aging
B. Irreversible damage has occurred by 24 hours.
C. It takes at least 48 hours for the active metabolite of methoxychlor to cause toxicity.
D. Oxines are not indicated in organochlorine insecticide toxicity.

1265. Methods to measure exposure to organophosphorus insecticides include _____.

A. red cell acetylcholinesterase
B. pseudocholinesterase in plasma
C. organophosphorus metabolites in urine
D. all of the above

1266. A syndrome of muscle weakness that occurs one to several days after acute poisoning with organophosphorus insecticides is called ____.

    A. nicotine syndrome
    B. intermediate syndrome
    C. organophosphate-induced delayed polyneuropathy
    D. serotonin syndrome

1267. The site of action for the toxicity of organophosphorus insecticides in causing organophosphorus-induced delayed polyneuropathy is ____.

    A. myelin
    B. nicotine receptor
    C. neuropathy target esterase
    D. cytochrome P450 2E1

1268. As a class, which of the following are most acutely toxic?

    A. insecticides
    B. rodenticides
    C. herbicides
    D. fungicides

1269. Worldwide, the highest percentage of poisoning deaths is due to ____.

    A. glyphosate and DEET
    B. triazines and alachlor
    C. paraquat and cholinesterase inhibitors
    D. rotenone and sodium fluoroacetate

1270. Which of the following is true of organophosphorus insecticides that contain a sulfur bound to phosphorus?

    A. They require bioactivation for activity.
    B. They are the most potent inhibitors of cytrochrome oxidase known.

C. There is no effective antidote.

D. The nerve gas sarin is an example.

1271. Which of the following is a carbamate insecticide?

A. metamidophos
B. diazinon
C. aldicarb
D. all of the above

1272. Carbamates differ from organophosphorus insecticides in that _____.

A. Cholinesterase inhibition is transient and reversible by carbamates.
B. Oxines are generally not used in carbamate poisonings.
C. Carbamylated acetylcholinesterase does not "age."
D. all of the above

1273. All of the following are true of pyrethrins except _____.

A. They have low mammalian toxicity.
B. They have high insecticidal potency.
C. They require bioactiviation.
D. They have low environmental persistence.

1274. The mode of action of pyrethroids is mediated through _____.

A. calcium channels
B. potassium channels
C. sodium channels
D. none of the above

1275. Type II pyrethroid insecticides differ from type 1 compounds in the presence of _____.

A. fluoride atoms
B. cyclopropyl groups

C. cyano groups

D. imidazole nucleus

1276. A distinguishing feature of type II pyrethroid toxicity in rats is the presence of _____.

A. behavioral arousal

B. clonic seizures

C. aggressive sparring

D. increased startle response

1277. The mechanism of toxicity of DDT is similar to that of _____.

A. allethrin

B. carbaryl

C. chlorpyrifos

D. malathion

1278. Lindane and cyclodiene insecticides have toxicity mediated through _____.

A. inhibition of cytrochrome P450

B. retinoic acid receptors

C. GABA receptor antagonism

D. increase in extracellular calcium

1279. All of the following are true of chlordecone except _____.

A. It causes tremors in humans.

B. It works by antagonism at the nicotine receptor.

C. It is excreted in the bile.

D. It is an inducer of P450.

1280. The mechanism of action of rotenone is _____.

A. blockade of sodium channels

B. stimulation of glutamate receptors

C. blockade of GABA receptors

D. inhibiting the mitochondrial respiratory chain

1281. All of the following are true of nicotine except _____.

A. Nicotine overdose both stimulates and paralyzes acetylcholine receptors.

B. Atropine is an antidote.

C. Dermal absorption could be significant.

D. Signs and symptoms of poisoning include nausea, vomiting, muscle weakness, and tachycardia.

1282. All of the following are true of neonicotinoids except _____.

A. Their use is increasing.

B. They are more selective for insect receptors than mammal receptors.

C. Their main drawback is that as a class, they are mutagenic.

D. Examples are imidacloprid and nitenpyram.

1283. All of the following are true of formanidines except _____.

A. Signs of poisoning include hypertension, tachycardia, and hypoglycemia.

B. Yohimbine is a theoretical antidote.

C. In invertebrates, they activate octopamine-dependent adenylate cyclase.

D. Amitraz is an example.

1284. All of the following are true of avermectins except _____.

A. They can be synthesized by a fungus.

B. They activate glutamate-dependent chloride channels in insects.

C. They can activate GABA receptors in vertebrates.

D. They are strong inhibitors of cytochrome P450 1A1.

1285. Piperonyl butoxide is added to increase the effect of _____.

   A. formamidines
   B. neonicotinoids
   C. pyrethroids
   D. avermectins

1286. Fipronil, a phenylpyrazole, acts by _____.

   A. blocking sodium channels
   B. stimulating glutamate receptor
   C. blocking picrotoxin-binding site used by organochlorines
   D. blocking GABA-gated chloride channel

1287. All of the following are true of Bacillus thuringienes except _____.

   A. It is classified as a biopesticide.
   B. It requires activation at pH less than 3.
   C. It is the most commonly used pesticide in its class.
   D. It has low mammalian toxicity.

1288. Citronella, DEET, and picaridin are classified as _____.

   A. insecticides
   B. herbicides
   C. insect repellents
   D. fungicides

1289. All of the following are true of 2, 4-D except _____.

   A. It is toxic to broad-leaved plants but not grasses.
   B. It is highly contaminated with TCDD.
   C. Urine alkalinization accelerates its clearance.
   D. It is extensively used throughout the world.

1290. All of the following are true of paraquat except _____.

    A. Most fatalities are secondary to dermal exposure.
    B. It may cause toxicity by redox cycling.
    C. Its target organs are lung and kidney.
    D. It is classified as a contact herbicide.

1291. All of the following are true of diquat except _____.

    A. It does not accumulate in the lung.
    B. It has some chemical similarity to paraquat.
    C. It is renal toxic.
    D. It is a human carcinogen.

1292. Chloroacetanilides _____.

    A. are rodenticides
    B. produce tumors at multiple locations in rats
    C. are associated with reproductive toxicity in humans
    D. include chlordimeform and amitraz as representative compounds

1293. Triazine herbicides _____.

    A. are classified as contact herbicides
    B. inhibit oxidative phosphorylation
    C. have low acute oral and dermal toxicity
    D. do not have a ring in their chemical structure

1294. All of the following are true of glyphosate except _____.

    A. It inhibits a metabolic pathway not present in mammals.
    B. It is widely used worldwide.
    C. It is selective for grasses over weeds.
    D. It has a phosphorus atom in its chemical structure.

1295. Captam and folpet are structurally similar to _____.

A. thalidomide
B. phencyclidine
C. morphine
D. urea

1296. All of the following are true of dithiocarbamates except
_____.

A. Maneb has been associated with Parkinson's disease.
B. They are structurally similar to disulfiram.
C. They are postemergent herbicides.
D. Some are associated with metal cations.

1297. The fungicide with the lowest toxicity is ____.

A. triphenyltin
B. copper sulfate
C. methylmercury
D. hexachlorobenzene

1298. All of the following are classified as rodenticides except
_____.

A. red squill
B. warfarin
C. glufosinate
D. sodium fluoroacetate

1299. Methyl bromide _____.

A. is an odorless gas
B. may deplete the ozone layer
C. is used as a fumigant
D. all of the above

Matching Test

1300. sarin

1301. fenvalerate

1302. 2, 4, 5-T

1303. acetochlor

1304. carbofuran

1305. propazine

1306. endrin

1307. thiram

1308. nithiazine

1309. benomyl

1310. chlorothalonil

1311. norbormide

1312. diquat

A.   rodenticide

B.   chlorphenoxy acid herbicide

C.   bipyridyl herbicide

D.   carbamate insecticide

E.   pyrethroid insecticide

F.   organochlorine insecticide

G.   dithiocarbamate fungicide

H.   neonicotinoid insecticide

I.   chloroacetanilide herbicide

J.   cholinesterase inhibitor

K.   triazine herbicide

L.   benzimidazole fungicide

M.   halogenated benzonitrile
       fungicide

CHAPTER 21 ANSWERS (REFERENCES)

1234. D (I)	1270. A (II)	1306. F (II)
1235. B (I)	1271. C (II)	1307. G (II)
1236. D (I)	1272. D (II)	1308. H (II)
1237. A (I)	1273. C (II)	1309. L (II)
1238. D (I)	1274. C (II)	1310. M (II)
1239. A (I)	1275. C (II)	1311. A (II)
1240. B (I)	1276. B (II)	1312. C (II)
1241. A (I)	1277. A (II)	
1242. C (I)	1278. C (II)	
1243. D (I)	1279. B (II)	
1244. A (I)	1280. D (II)	
1245. B (I)	1281. B (II)	
1246. C (I)	1282. C (II)	
1247. A (I)	1283. A (II)	
1248. C (II)	1284. D (II)	
1249. B (II)	1285. C (II)	
1250. A (II)	1286. D (II)	
1251. D (II)	1287. B (II)	
1252. B (II)	1288. C (II)	
1253. D (II)	1289. B (II)	
1254. B (II)	1290. A (II)	
1255. B (II)	1291. D (II)	
1256. C (II)	1292. B (II)	
1257. D (II)	1293. C (II)	
1258. B (III)	1294. C (II)	
1259. D (III)	1295. A (II)	
1260. A (III)	1296. C (II)	
1261. B (III)	1297. B (II)	
1262. C (III)	1298. C (II)	
1263. C (II)	1299. D (II)	
1264. D (II)	1300. J (II)	
1265. D (II)	1301. E (II)	
1266. B (II)	1302. B (II)	
1267. C (II)	1303. I (II)	
1268. A (II)	1304. D (II)	
1269. C (II)	1305. K (II)	

REFERENCES

CHAPTER 21

I.   M. A. O'Malley, "Pesticides," in *Current Occupational and Environmental Medicine*, 4th ed., ed. J. Landou (New York: McGraw-Hill, 2007), 532–578.

II.   L. G., Costa, "Toxic Effects of Pesticides," in *Casarett & Doull's Toxicology: The Basic Science of Poisons*, 7th ed., ed. C.D. Klaassen (New York: McGraw-Hill, 2008), 883–930.

III. C. B. Breckenridge and J. T. Stevens, "Crop Protection Chemicals: Mechanisms of Action and Hazard Profiles," in *Principles and Methods of Toxicology*, 5th ed., ed. A.W. Hayes (Boca Raton: Taylor and Francis, 2008), 727–840.

22

ANIMAL TOXICOLOGY

1313. The larger macromolecules of snake venom are probably _____.

   A. transported by OAT
   B. broken down by enzymes in the subcutaneous tissue to small components
   C. never absorbed but act locally
   D. absorbed through the lymphatics

1314. Toxins produced by poisonous animals usually are derived _____.

   A. from photochemical reactions
   B. from altered purine and pyrimidine synthesis
   C. from the food chain
   D. from chemicals in the soil and water

1315. Envenomation from *Centruroides* genus of scorpion in children produces _____.

   A. nystagmus, tachycardia, fasciculations
   B. bradycardia, dry mouth, hypothermia
   C. fever, sweating, dilated pupils
   D. blindness, polyuria, jaundice

1316. The ω-agatoxins have selectivity for vertebrae _____.

    A. calcium channels
    B. potassium channels
    C. sodium channels
    D. chloride channels

1317. The spider genus that causes the longest pain duration after biting a human is _____.

    A. *Steatoda*
    B. *Lamponidae*
    C. *Loxosceles*
    D. *Latrodectus*

1318. Which of the following genus of spiders produces a skin lesion up to 10 cm wide with muscle invasion and necrosis after envenomation?

    A. *Loxosceles*
    B. *Agelenopsis*
    C. *Latrodectus*
    D. *Theraphosidae*

1319. All of the following are true of tarantula bites except _____.

    A. Death occurs in 10 % of cases.
    B. Cramps and muscle spasms can occur.
    C. The venom contains peptides.
    D. Local pain, itching, and tenderness can occur.

1320. All of the following are true of ticks except _____.

    A. The saliva contains toxins.
    B. They will suck blood from a victim for 24 hours or more before injecting saliva.
    C. The bite is often not felt.
    D. Skin lesions may not appear until several days after the bite.

1321. Centipede bites _____.

    A. cause seizures
    B. produce pulmonary toxicity
    C. release a cardiac toxin that mimics cholinergic stimulation
    D. can cause liver failure

1322. Eye injuries can result from toxins sprayed by

    A. brown recluse spiders
    B. centipedes
    C. scorpions
    D. millipedes

1323. All of the following are frog and/or toad toxins except _____.

    A. saxitoxin
    B. bufotoxin
    C. batrachotoxin
    D. histrionicotoxin

1324. Three of the following animals produce a venom with similar effects. The animal with a venom that has a different mechanism of action is _____.

    A. rattlesnake
    B. salamander
    C. water moccasin
    D. copperhead

1325. The toxin of the pufferfish concentrates in _____.

    A. brain and nerves
    B. heart and skeletal muscle
    C. liver and ovaries
    D. kidney and eye

1326. The toxin in the pufferfish causes death by _____.

    A. hyperthermia
    B. pulmonary edema
    C. respiratory paralysis
    D. liver failure

1327. The toxin from the sea snake _____.

    A. is one of the most potent vertebrate toxins
    B. is only harmful to animals
    C. is a mixture of non-proteins
    D. none of the above

1328. All of the following are true of the Portuguese man-of-war (Physalia physalis) except _____.

    A. An effective antivenom exists.
    B. Death can occur from stings.
    C. Acetic acid has no effect on relief of symptoms.
    D. Topical lidocaine can be used to reduce pain.

1329. All of the following are true of sea urchins except _____.

    A. Most urchins cannot inject venom into humans.
    B. Two species from the Pacific Ocean can inflict serious envenomations.
    C. They are in the phylum Mollusca.
    D. Most stings from urchins result in primarily mechanical injuries.

1330. All of the following types of bony fish are toxin-producing except _____.

    A. boxfish
    B. rabbitfish
    C. scorpion fish
    D. koi

1331. All of the following snakes release significant neurotoxins except _____.

A. Eastern diamond-backed rattlesnake
B. coral
C. cobra
D. mamba

1332. The alkaloid toxins of several brightly colored poison dart frogs come from _____.

A. photochemical reactions in their skin
B. a diet of certain ants
C. swimming in collections of toxic algae
D. a diet of seeds containing cyanide

1333. A coagulopathy could result from envenomation from certain species of South American _____.

A. spiders
B. moths
C. scorpions
D. ants

1334. Nondisulfide-rich conpeptides target all of the following receptors except _____.

A. opiate
B. vasopression
C. NMDA
D. neurotensin

1335. The disulfide-rich conopeptides target all of the following ion channels except _____.

A. sodium
B. potassium
C. phosphate
D. calcium

1336. All of the following are true regarding snakes except _____.

    A. Most chew their food before swallowing it.
    B. Pit vipers can sense warm-blooded animals.
    C. The Colubridae is the largest venomous family.
    D. The Viperidae fang is a highly efficient structure for toxin delivery.

1337. Sarafotoxins present in asps of Afro-Arabia can cause _____.

    A. hepatic vein thrombosis
    B. common bile duct stones
    C. bronchiolitis obliterans
    D. coronary artery constriction

1338. All of the following statements are true regarding animal toxins except _____.

    A. Some venoms can contain more than 100 proteins.
    B. Venoms can be used to study normal physiology.
    C. Snake toxins are usually more potent than botulinum toxin.
    D. Some venoms have been a source of marketed drugs.

1339. All of the following statements are true of scorpion venoms except _____.

    A. They can affect potassium channels.
    B. The major neurotoxins are nonpeptides.
    C. They can affect sodium channels.
    D. Not all scorpions have toxins that affect neurotrans-mission.

1340. A significant toxin associated with black widow spiders is _____.

    A. alpha-latrotoxin
    B. alpha-cobrotoxin

C. batrachotoxin
D. ciguatoxin

1341. Ticks are associated with all of the following except _____.

A. Lyme disease
B. paralysis
C. methicillin-resistant staph
D. babesiosis

1342. Bites from centipedes are unusual in that _____.

A. They are painless.
B. They cause black streaking.
C. They have delayed toxicity 1 week later.
D. They produce 2 small punctures.

1343. An important component of ant venom is _____.

A. sodium hydroxide
B. formic acid
C. phenols
D. potassium ions

1344. An unusual aspect of cone snail toxin is _____.

A. Sometimes the toxin can kill the cone snail.
B. It is only 1 toxin.
C. Varying ocean temperatures will lead to different toxins.
D. Multiple toxins act synergistically.

1345. The venom from the Gila monster _____.

A. does not have a commercially available antivenom
B. is similar to the coral snake
C. is a frequent cause of death
D. is used in cancer treatments

1346. All of the following statements are true of rattlesnake venom except _____.

  A. The venoms are usually complex mixture.
  B. They usually affect integrity of blood vessels and coagulation mechanisms.
  C. They are all strongly neurotoxic.
  D. Hypotension can be a life-threatening outcome.

1347. Antivenoms _____.

  A. can be produced against snake, spider, and scorpion toxins
  B. can be monovalent or polyvalent
  C. can cause type I or type III hypersensitivity reactions
  D. all of the above

1348. Cobra venom factor _____.

  A. stimulates nicotinic acetycholine receptors
  B. activates the complement cascade
  C. stimulates glutamate receptors
  D. none of the above

1349. Drug useful in the treatment of hypertension (angiotensin converting enzyme inhibitors) have been developed from_____.

  A. scorpion venom
  B. wasp venom
  C. brown recluse spider venom
  D. venom from Bothrops jararaca (pit viper)

Matching Test

1350. sea turtle

    A. more toxic species than any other genus in animal kingdom

1351. leech

    B. venom contains tetrodotoxin and hapalotoxin

1352. anemone

    C. venomous starfish

1353. crown of thorns

    D. venom contains solenopsins

1354. lionfish

    E. TTX present in the skin of some species

1355. boxfish

    F. venom similar to Gila Monster

1356. cone snail

    G. targets Ca^{+2} ion channel

1357. blue-ringed octopus

    H. targets acetylcholinesterase

1358. fire ant

    I. targets K^+ ion channel

1359. beaded lizard

    J. targets cell membrane

1360. frogs

    K. algal toxins accumulate in meat

1361. draculin

    L. targets Na^{+1} ion channel

1362. phospholipase A2

    M. anticoagulant

1363. dendrotoxin

    N. aquarium fish that releases toxin into environment

1364. omega-agatoxin

    O. aquarium fish that contains venom on spines

1365. tetrodotoxin

    P. contains actinosporins

1366. fasciculin

    Q. depletes blood volume in small animals

CHAPTER 22 ANSWERS (REFERENCES)

1313.	D (I)		1349.	D (I)
1314.	C (I)		1350.	K (II)
1315.	A (I)		1351.	Q (II)
1316.	A (I)		1352.	P (II)
1317.	D (I)		1353.	C (II)
1318.	A (I)		1354.	O (II)
1319.	A (I)		1355.	N (II)
1320.	B (I)		1356.	A (II)
1321.	C (I)		1357.	B (II)
1322.	D (I)		1358.	D (II)
1323.	A (II)		1359.	F (II)
1324.	B (II)		1360.	E (II)
1325.	C (II)		1361.	M (II)
1326.	C (II)		1362.	J (II)
1327.	A (II)		1363.	I (II)
1328.	A (II)		1364.	G (II)
1329.	C (II)		1365.	L (II)
1330.	D (II)		1366.	H (II)
1331.	A (II)			
1332.	B (II)			
1333.	B (I)			
1334.	A (I)			
1335.	C (I)			
1336.	A (I)			
1337.	D (I)			
1338.	C (I)			
1339.	B (I)			
1340.	A (I)			
1341.	C (I)			
1342.	D (I)			
1343.	B (I)			
1344.	D (I)			
1345.	A (I)			
1346.	C (I)			
1347.	D (I)			
1348.	B (I)			

REFERENCES

CHAPTER 22

I.   J. B. Watkins, "Properties and Toxicities of Animal Venoms," in *Casarett & Doull's Toxicology: The Basic Science of Poisons*, 7th ed., ed. C. D. Klaassen (New York: McGraw-Hill, 2008),1083–1102.

II.   F. W. Oehme and D. E. Keyler, "Plant and Animal Toxins," in *Principles and Methods of Toxicology*, 5th ed., ed. A.W. Hayes (Boca Raton: Taylor and Francis, 2008), 983–1054.

23

TOXICOLOGY OF PLANTS

1367. *Euphorbia marginata* (snow-on-the-mountain) causes contact dermatitis by excreting _____.

A. phenols
B. benzaldehyde
C. fatty acids
D. latex

1368. In *Rhus radicans* (poison ivy), the contact allergen is _____.

A. urushiol
B. capsaicin
C. usnic acid
D. ergot

1369. The most common event that usually occurs from ingestion of a toxic plant is _____.

A. asthma
B. nausea, vomiting, diarrhea
C. skin rash
D. mental confusion

1370. Saint Anthony's fire is due to the ingestion of _____.

A. mushrooms
B. ricin

C. ergot alkaloids
D. wisteria

1371. A toxin that increases the cough reflex is _____.

A. pyrrolizidine alkaloids
B. brucine
C. caulophylline
D. capsaicin

1372. A toxin produced in the poppy plant that intercalates DNA is _____.

A. ptaquiloside
B. sanguinarine
C. silymarin
D. ochratoxin A

1373. The false morel mushroom *Gyromitra esculenta* has been associated with _____.

A. leukemia
B. gangrene
C. hepatitis
D. increased cardiac contractions

1374. The mechanisms of action of ricin is _____.

A. inhibition of protein synthesis
B. uncoupling of oxidative phosphorylation
C. increasing intracellular calcium
D. activation of proto-oncogenes

1375. Mad honey poisoning is due to _____.

A. grayanotoxin
B. convallatoxin
C. pyrrolizidine alkaloids
D. 4-ipomeanol

1376. Cascara sagrada has medicinal use as _____.

    A. an antidepressant
    B. a laxative
    C. a phytoestrogen
    D. an antidiarrheal

1377. The alkaloids in *Symphytum* cause a human condition that resembles _____.

    A. Pott's disease
    B. toxic shock syndrome
    C. Addison's disease
    D. Budd-Chiari syndrome

1378. In cattle, ingestion of *Lantana camara* (Verbenaceae) causes _____.

    A. cholestasis
    B. abortions
    C. abnormal behavior
    D. renal failure

1379. Veratrum alkaloids cause _____.

    A. hepatitis
    B. bradycardia
    C. bladder tumors
    D. lung fibrosis

1380. Squill and lily of the valley contain _____.

    A. pyrrolizidine alkaloids
    B. teratogens
    C. cardiac glycosides
    D. inner ear toxins

1381. American mistletoe contains _____.

    A. jervine
    B. phoratoxin
    C. abrin-a
    D. aconitine

1382. Datura species of houseplants contain _____.

    A. strychnine
    B. muscarinic agents
    C. anticholinergic agents
    D. sympathomimetic agents

1383. A toxic ingredient in locoweed is _____.

    A. atropine
    B. domoic acid
    C. ibotenic acid
    D. swainsonine

1384. All of the following are excitatory amino acids except _____.

    A. jervine
    B. domoic acid
    C. ibotenic acid
    D. willardine

1385. Seizures have been associated with all of the following except _____.

    A. parsley family of plants
    B. spurge family of plants
    C. mint family of plants
    D. species of *Strychnos*

1386. Dicumarol is a fungal metabolite that causes _____.

A. arrhythmias
B. seizures
C. hallucinations
D. bleeding

1387. Lysergic acid derivatives are produced by _____.

A. *Amanita* mushrooms
B. *Gyromitra* mushrooms
C. *Fusarium* fungus
D. *Acremonium* fungus

1388. Ochratoxin is a/an _____.

A. positive ionotropic agent
B. immunosuppressant
C. lung toxin
D. cholinergic agent

1389. Linamarin is a/an _____.

A. pyrrolizidine alkaloid
B. cardioactive glycoside
C. cyanogenic glucoside
D. fungal metabolite

1390. Motor neuron demyelination results from ingestion of _____.

A. cassava
B. *Strychnos* genus
C. linamarin
D. anthracenones

1391. All of the following contain anticholinergic alkaloids except
_____.

A. henbane
B. oleander
C. deadly nightshade
D. jimsonweed

1392. Aconitine causes toxicity by _____.

A. stimulating GABA receptors
B. opening up calcium channels
C. prolonging sodium current in cardiac muscle
D. inhibiting glycine receptors

1393. Taxol is present in _____.

A. autumn crocus
B. Western yew
C. glory lily
D. mayapple

1394. A toxin present in potatoes and tomatoes is _____.

A. colchicine
B. vinblastine
C. solanine
D. podophyllotoxin

1395. Abrin mechanistically most resembles _____.

A. ricin
B. linamarin
C. caulophylline
D. scopolamine

1396. Methyllycaconitine mechanistically most resembles _____.

    A. physostigmine
    B. digitalis
    C. atropine
    D. curare

1397. Monomethylhydrazine is found in _____.

    A. algae
    B. lichens
    C. ferns
    D. mushrooms

1398. Psilocybin is known to mostly affect which brain receptor?

    A. norepinephrine
    B. dopamine
    C. GABA
    D. serotonin

1399. Rhubarb, mother-in-law's tongue, and philodendron all contain _____.

    A. oxalate
    B. cyanide
    C. nicotine
    D. atropine

1400. Microcystin's mechanism of action may be _____.

    A. biliary statis
    B. portal vein thrombosis
    C. destruction of liver cytoskeleton
    D. T cell mediated

1401. Uncooked, wild, "nontoxic" mushrooms can be toxic to _____.

 A. adults
 B. children
 C. diabetics
 D. asthmatics

1402. The least common toxicity from plant ingestion is _____.

 A. hepatic toxicity
 B. pancreatic toxicity
 C. cardiac toxicity
 D. dermatitis

1403. All of the following are made by plants except _____.

 A. opiates
 B. cocaine
 C. benzodiazepines
 D. hallucinogens

1404. Which of the following chemical classes is least likely to be a plant toxin?

 A. alcohols
 B. alkaloids
 C. glycosides
 D. hydrocarbons

1405. Ingestion of daffodil bulbs would first produce _____.

 A. gastrointestinal symptoms
 B. cardiac symptoms
 C. neurologic symptoms
 D. photosensitivity

1406. Dumbcane contains oxalate which acts as a _____.

    A. neurotoxin
    B. cardiac toxin
    C. hematologic toxin
    D. mucus membrane contact irritant

1407. Physostigmine would be considered as an antidote for ingestion of _____.

    A. crocus
    B. water hemlock
    C. angel's trumpet
    D. locoweed

1408. Ergovaline inhibits _____.

    A. insulin release
    B. prolactin release
    C. vasopressin release
    D. aldosterone release

1409. An abortifacient present in tropical legumes is _____.

    A. mimosine
    B. anagyrine
    C. thermopsine
    D. jervine

1410. Which of the following findings would be least likely to be found as a primary disease in a person who ingested Amanita phalloides?

    A. liver pathology
    B. brain pathology
    C. kidney pathology
    D. intestinal pathology

1411. All of the following are manifestations of belladonna alkaloid poisoning except _____.

    A. dry mouth
    B. dilated pupils
    C. hallucinations
    D. bronchospasm

1412. Cattle-consuming *Solanum malacoxylon* (Solanocene) develop a disease similar to _____.

    A. Parkinson's disease
    B. Addison's disease
    C. vitamin D intoxication
    D. SIADH

1413. The mechanism of action of podophyllotoxin is similar to that of _____.

    A. ricin
    B. rotenone
    C. colchicine
    D. ouabain

1414. Ricin comes from _____.

    A. lily of the valley
    B. castor bean plant
    C. oleander
    D. wisteria

1415. All of the following produce alkaloids that affect the heart except _____.

    A. European hellebore
    B. monkshood
    C. petunia
    D. rhododendron

1416. Saint Anthony's fire is produced by _____.

    A. arsenic
    B. *Claviceps purpurea*
    C. false morel mushrooms
    D. *Lantana camara*

1417. Pyrrolizidine alkaloids are associated with _____.

    A. heptic veno-occlusive disease
    B. hallucinations
    C. renal failure
    D. all of the above

1418. All of the following contribute to the variability in toxin produced by a plant except _____.

    A. varying toxin concentration in different parts of plant
    B. age of the plant
    C. climate and soil
    D. type of local herbivore

1419. A cross sensitivity between individuals allergic to latex gloves and some plant components is known as _____.

    A. latex-root syndrome
    B. latex-leaf syndrome
    C. latex-fruit syndrome
    D. latex-seed syndrome

1420. A potential human hepatotoxin produce by lichens is _____.

    A. domoic acid
    B. usnic acid
    C. butytric acid
    D. carbolic acid

1421. Saint John's wort can cause which of the following in sheep
_____.

A. photosensitivity
B. infertility
C. renal failure
D. abnormal behavior

1422. 4-ipomeanol causes which type of toxicity in animals?

A. liver and pancreatic
B. lung and renal
C. heart and muscle
D. neurologic

1423. Most fatal mushroom poisoning occurs from all of the following
genera except _____.

A. *Amanita*
B. *Gyromitra*
C. *Galerina*
D. *Lepiota*

1424. Alpha-amanitian _____.

A. is responsible for the diarrhea seen in death cap poisoning
B. is poorly absorbed orally
C. is a potent inhibitor of hepatic protein synthesis
D. none of the above

1425. Aflatoxins are dangerous to human because they _____.

A. are present in wet basements
B. cause pneumonia in AIDS patients
C. are associated with nasal carcinoma
D. none of the above

1426. Which of the following plants is carcinogenic?

A. American hellebore
B. bracken fern
C. buttercup
D. tung nut

1427. All of the following are true of grayanotoxins except _____.

A. They are present in rhododendron.
B. They can contaminate honey.
C. They cause bradycardia.
D. They block the neuromuscular junction.

1428. Plant molecules that react as bases and usually contain nitrogen in a heterocyclic structure are known as _____.

A. alkaloids
B. terpenes
C. resins
D. glycosides

1429. Plant molecules that are created from isoprene units with varying functional groups are known as _____.

A. terpenes
B. amines
C. alkaloids
D. phenols

1430. Plant molecules that are hydrolyzed to a sugar and a nonsugar moiety are known as _____.

A. glycosides
B. alkaloids
C. resins
D. terpene

1431. Toxic minerals that may accumulate in plants include all of the following except _____.

A. cadmium
B. magnesium
C. copper
D. selenium

1432. *Brassica oleracea* (kale) contains a _____.

A. cardiac glycoside
B. cyanogenic glycoside
C. goiterogenic glycoside
D. steroid glycoside

1433. A plant toxin that can be highly transmitted through milk is _____.

A. oxalate
B. cyanide
C. nitrate
D. tremetol

1434. An antidote is available for the toxin present in _____.

A. azalea
B. pigweed
C. veratrum
D. apple seeds

1435. Which of the following plant toxins is classified as an alcohol?

A. nicotine
B. ranunculus
C. dogbane
D. tremetol

1436. Amygdalin is found in the highest amounts in the seeds of
_____.

A. bitter almond
B. tomato
C. pear
D. plum

1437. Strychnine blocks _____.

A. glycine-gated chloride channel
B. glutamate receptors
C. GABA receptors
D. voltage-gated sodium channels

1438. The toxin found in species of Capsicum has been shown to be
useful in the therapy of _____.

A. skin cancer
B. depression
C. chronic pain
D. decubitus ulcers

1439. All of the following are true of curare except _____.

A. It was a South American arrow poison.
B. It is a neuromuscular blocking agent.
C. It can be used clinically.
D. It is CNS toxic.

1440. Swainsonine _____.

A. is present in vinca species
B. is a glycoprotein
C. causes abortions in livestock
D. none of the above

1441. The veratrum and lupine alkaloids are _____.

    A. teratogenic
    B. components of marketed pharmaceuticals
    C. used as insecticides
    D. poisons that Socrates drank

Matching Test

1442. apricot   A. anticholinergic

1443. water hemlock   B. nausea, vomiting

1444. lupine   C. soluble oxalate

1445. cactus   D. seizures, tremors

1446. poinsettia   E. CNS cognitive

1447. oleander   F. photosensitivity-inducing

1448. jimsonweed   G. cyanide

1449. Saint-John's-wort   H. contact irritant dermatitis

1450. rhubarb   I. hepatotoxic and teratogenic

1451. marijuana   J. cardiac arrhythmias

CHAPTER 23 ANSWERS (REFERENCES)

1367. D (I)	1403. C (II)	1439. D (I)
1368. A (I)	1404. D (II)	1440. C (I)
1369. B (I)	1405. A (II)	1441. A (I)
1370. C (I)	1406. D (II)	1442. G (II)
1371. D (I)	1407. C (I)	1443. D (II)
1372. B (I)	1408. B (I)	1444. I (II)
1373. C (I)	1409. A (I)	1445. H (II)
1374. A (I)	1410. B (I)	1446. B (II)
1375. A (I)	1411. D (I)	1447. J (II)
1376. B (I)	1412. C (I)	1448. A (II)
1377. D (I)	1413. C (I)	1449. F (II)
1378. A (I)	1414. B (I)	1450. C (II)
1379. B (I)	1415. C (I)	1451. E (II)
1380. C (I)	1416. B (I)	
1381. B (I)	1417. A (I)	
1382. C (I)	1418. D (I)	
1383. D (I)	1419. C (I)	
1384. A (I)	1420. B (I)	
1385. B (I)	1421. A (I)	
1386. D (I)	1422. B (I)	
1387. D (I)	1423. B (I)	
1388. B (I)	1424. C (I)	
1389. C (I)	1425. D (I)	
1390. D (I)	1426. B (I)	
1391. B (I)	1427. D (I)	
1392. C (I)	1428. A (III)	
1393. B (I)	1429. A (III)	
1394. C (I)	1430. A (III)	
1395. A (I)	1431. B (II)	
1396. D (I)	1432. C (II)	
1397. D (II)	1433. D (II)	
1398. D (II)	1434. D (II)	
1399. A (II)	1435. D (II)	
1400. C (II)	1436. A (I)	
1401. B (II)	1437. A (I)	
1402. B (II)	1438. C (I)	

REFERENCES

CHAPTER 23

I. S. Norton, "Toxic Effects of Plants," in *Casarett & Doull's Toxicology: The Basic Science of Poisons*, 7th ed., C. D. Klaassen (New York: McGraw-Hill, 2008), 1103–1116.

II. F. W. Oehme and D. E. Keyler, "Plant and Animal Toxins," in *Principles and Methods of Toxicology*, 5th ed., ed. A. W. Hayes (Boca Raton: CRC Press, 2008), 984–1052.

III. M. E. Palmer and J. M. Betz, "Plants," in *Goldfrank's Toxicologic Emergencies*, 9th ed., ed. L. S. Nelson et al. (New York: McGraw-Hill, 2011), 1537–1560.

24

RADIATION TOXICOLOGY

1452. The most frequent types of DNA damage in mammalian cells produced by low LET radiation exposure are _____.

A. double-strand breaks
B. single-strand breaks
C. DNA protein cross-links
D. DNA dimers

1453. Beta particles are emitted with a continuous energy spectum because of the simultaneous emission of a/an _____.

A. protein
B. gamma ray
C. X-ray
D. antineutrino

1454. An example of a pure gamma ray emitter is _____.

A. technetium 99m
B. carbon 14
C. sodium 22
D. oxygen 16

1455. Photons interact with matter in all of the following ways except
_____.

A. pair production
B. dark energy production
C. photoelectric effect
D. Compton effect

1456. Internal conversion produces _____.

A. an atom without an orbital electron
B. an atom of higher atomic number
C. an atom of lower atomic number
D. an electron from a gamma ray

1457. If a photon possesses energy of the order 1.02 MeV, it is capable
of _____.

A. splitting a helium nucleus
B. producing a positron and electron
C. converting a neutron into a proton and electron
D. creating an alpha particle

1458. Which of the following has the least ability to penetrate the
skin?

A. beta particle
B. neutron
C. X-ray
D. gamma rays

1459. Alpha particles are most dangerous when they _____.

A. do not have relativistic velocities
B. are produced from helium
C. are inhaled
D. are in contact with the skin

1460. The biological effects of radiation are due to all of the following except _____.

A. breaking hydrogen bonds
B. free radical formation
C. breaking covalent bonds
D. forming coordination complexes with biological metals

1461. Combination of an inner-shell electron with a nuclear proton is called_____.

A. electron capture
B. positron emission
C. beta-decay
D. none of the above

1462. The occupation guidelines for radiation protection developed in a 1990 document by the Internal Commission on Radiation Protection are _____.

A. 100mSv in 5 years
B. 250mSv in 5 years
C. 500mSv in 5 years
D. 1Sv in 5 years

1463. Much of the DNA damage from high LET (linear energy transfer) radiation _____.

A. is readily repairable
B. results from localized clusters of ionization
C. occurs in many cells along a tract receiving a small dose
D. all of the above

1464. The late health effect of radium ingestion in radium dial painters was _____.

A. acute myelogenous leukemia
B. aplastic anemia

C. osteogenic sarcoma

D. multiple myeloma

1465. Children under 18 at the time of the Chernobyl nuclear accident developed the greatest increase in incidence of _____.

A. lung cancer

B. liver cancer

C. thyroid cancer

D. colon cancer

1466. The lung cancer risk in uranium miners is due to _____.

A. uranium 234

B. lead 214

C. radon 226 and its decay products

D. thorium 234

1467. All of the following are true of indoor radon exposure except _____.

A. Open flames in a house produce a higher exposure.

B. Urban areas have the same radon levels as rural areas.

C. Smokers have a higher risk per unit of exposure.

D. Particle size can change the dose delivered to the lungs.

1468. The largest percentage of natural background radiation that the human body receives is from _____.

A. short-lived daughter isotopes of radon

B. cosmic rays

C. medical X-rays

D. dietary intake of potassium 40

1469. The largest amount of terrestrial background radiation comes from _____.

A. nitrogen, oxygen, and silicon

B. plutonium, thallium, and technetium

C. sodium, potassium, and cesium

D. uranium, thorium, and potassium

1470. A process that creates the same product nuclei as position emission is _____.

A. alpha decay

B. gamma ray production

C. electron capture

D. beta decay

1471. The characteristic of alpha particles which causes a high energy loss per path length and a high ionization density along the track length is called _____.

A. high Compton effect

B. high linear energy transfer

C. high photoelectric effect

D. high energy pair production

1472. Beta particles moving near the speed of light _____.

A. have a wavelength in the visible range

B. rarely interact with matter

C. must have relativistic effects applied to them

D. frequently decompose into gamma rays and neutrinos

1473. The unit of absorbed dose for ionizing radiation is _____.

A. rem

B. sievert (Sv)

C. roentgen

D. gray (Gy)

1474. The unit of equivalent dose for ionizing radiation is _____.

A. rem

B. sievert (Sv)

C. roentgen

D. gray (Gy)

1475. The term-effective dose of ionizing radiation _____.

A. is a dose that causes necrosis of particular cell types

B. is the equivalent dose divided by the weight of body tissue

C. allows for a direct comparison of the cancer risk from different partial or whole-body doses

D. is a dose that kills greater than 99 % of malignant cells in a particular tissue

CHAPTER 24 ANSWERS (REFERENCES)

1452. B (I)
1453. D (I)
1454. A (I)
1455. B (I)
1456. A (I)
1457. B (I)
1458. A (II)
1459. C (II)
1460. D (III)
1461. A (I)
1462. A (I)
1463. B (I)
1464. C (I)
1465. C (I)
1466. C (I)
1467. B (I)
1468. A (I)
1469. D (I)
1470. C (I)
1471. B (I)
1472. C (I)
1473. D (I)
1474. B (I)
1475. C (I)

REFERENCES

CHAPTER 24

I. N. H. Harley, "Health Effects of Radiation and Radioactive Materials," in *Casarett & Doull's Toxicology: The Basic Science of Poisons*, 7th ed., ed. C. D. Klaassen (New York: McGraw-Hill, 2008),1053–1082.

II. R. Cohen and S. Horie, "Injuries Caused by Physical Hazards," in *Current Occupational and Environmental Medicine*, 4th ed., ed. J. Landou (New York: McGraw-Hill, 2007), 122–150.

III. L. G. Cockerham et al., "Ionizing Radiation," in *Principles and Methods of Toxicology*, 5th ed., ed. J. Landou (Boca Raton: Taylor and Francis, 2008), 897–982.

25

ENVIRONMENTAL TOXICOLOGY

1476. The concentration of chemical in an organism divided by the concentration of chemical in the water in which the organism comes in contact with is called _____.

   A. biota sediment accumulation factor
   B. organism/water partition coefficient
   C. food chain ratio
   D. bioconcentration factor

1477. Biomanification is a/an _____.

   A. increase in chemical concentration in animal tissue compared to surrounding water
   B. increase in chemical concentration in an organism as it moves up the food chain
   C. increase in unionized form of chemical as it enters an organism
   D. sudden availability of previously sequestered chemicals in an organism

1478. In a body of water, the insoluble form of a metal is usually in the form of a/an _____.

   A. chlorate
   B. sulfate
   C. sulfide
   D. bromide

1479. All of the following biotransformation enzymes are upregulated by ligand binding to the AH (aryl hydrocarbon) receptor except _____.

A. CYP1A1
B. CYP2E1
C. CYP1A2
D. CYP1B1

1480. The earthworm survival test is used to test the toxicity of _____.

A. river water
B. rainwater
C. soil
D. groundwater

1481. Lichens are useful to test for the effects of _____.

A. air pollution
B. endocrine disrupters
C. radiation
D. oil spills

1482. All of the following are true of water-soluble toxicants compared to more lipid-soluble toxicants except _____.

A. They disperse more in the environment.
B. They are less sorbed to soil.
C. They are less sorbed to sediments.
D. They bioaccumulate.

1483. Biodegradation of toxicants in the environment occurs primarily by _____.

A. mammalian liver metabolism
B. photochemical reactors
C. microbial metabolism
D. chemical reactions on limestone

1484. The most common screening test for environmental chemicals is _____.

A. acute toxicity
B. repeat-dose toxicity
C. carcinogenicity
D. reproductive toxicity

1485. In a community, the keystone species is _____.

A. the population with the largest number
B. the population that has a crucial role
C. the population most sensitive to toxicants
D. the population in danger of extinction

1486. The richness of a community is _____.

A. the number of different species
B. the number of different genera
C. the ratio of the number of animal species to number of plant species
D. the number of keystone species

1487. Evenness of a community refers to _____.

A. the ratio of keystone species to dominate species
B. the ratio of predators to prey
C. the ratio of carnivores to herbivores
D. how equitably the individuals in a community are spread among the species

1488. IBI stands for _____.

A. Institute of Biotic Information
B. Index of Biological Identity
C. Index of Biotic Integrity
D. Inorganic Biotic Identity

1489. Which of the following would be considered a biomarker?

   A. concentration of methylmercury in river water
   B. pH of acid rain
   C. concentration of PAH-DNA adducts
   D. number of pregnant rainbow trout

1490. An example of a chemical producing an adverse effect on an animal's immune function is _____.

   A. pesticides in amphibians
   B. PCBs in channel catfish
   C. heavy metals in rainbow trout
   D. all of the above

1491. Organophosphate insecticide and methylmercury exposures have had a major impact on wildlife _____.

   A. cardiac development
   B. liver development
   C. kidney development
   D. behavior

1492. Cancer associated with chemical contaminates of aquatic systems is highest in _____.

   A. species that live close to the surface
   B. species that eat plankton
   C. species that live in sediments
   D. species that eat shrimp

1493. A collection of members of the same species that occupy the same location and within which can exchange genetic information is called a _____.

   A. genus
   B. population
   C. subpopulation
   D. community

1494. All of the following factors can reduce population densities except _____.

   A. argon levels
   B. toxicant exposure
   C. weather
   D. number of predators

1495. Toxicants added to aquatic systems that enhance the growth of phytoplankton can cause fish and invertebrate mortality by _____.

   A. lowered nitrate levels
   B. competition for sunlight
   C. hypoxia
   D. attraction of predators

1496. Organochlorine pesticides affect avian reproduction by causing _____.

   A. maternal hypertension
   B. eggshell thinning
   C. decreased ovulation
   D. abruptio placentae

1497. Morpholinos are used to _____.

   A. transiently block translation of specific proteins
   B. block oxidative phosphorylation
   C. enhance translation of specific proteins
   D. repair DNA damage

1498. Developmental effects in fish embryos have been associated with all of the following except _____.

   A. increased particulate matter in the air
   B. oil spills
   C. paper mill effluents
   D. creosote

1499. Stimulation of CYP1A1 in zebra fish _____.

    A. provides some protection against embryo toxicity for carcinogens that are metabolized to less-toxic compounds
    B. provide some protection against dioxin-mediated embryo toxicity
    C. enhances the toxicity of reactive nitrogen species
    D. all of the above

1500. All of the following act as AHR ligands except _____.

    A. bisphenol A
    B. dioxin
    C. benzopyrene
    D. 3-methylcholanthrene

1501. A liver enzyme that is a marker for vertebrae exposure to inducers of AHR is _____.

    A. vitellogenin
    B. alkaline phosphase
    C. aspartate transaminase
    D. ethoxyresorufin-O-deethylase (EROD)

1502. Birds exposed to spent lead shot will have inhibition of _____.

    A. acetylcholinesterase
    B. ALAD
    C. CYP2E1
    D. AST

1503. The effects of pollutants on mitochondrial energy metabolism can be particularly devastating to wildlife because _____.

    A. Certain species have fewer mitochondria per cell as compared to those of humans.
    B. Certain species have less-efficient oxidative phosphorylation as compared to that of humans.

C. Food sources are depleted during the winter.

D. They have less brown fat than humans do.

1504. PAHs, metals, and nanoparticles can be sequestered in _____.

A. mitochondria

B. ribosomes

C. endoplasmic reticulum

D. lysosomes

1505. Increased vitellogenin levels in male fish are a biomarker for _____.

A. xenoestrogen exposure

B. polyaromatic hydrocarbon exposure

C. oxidative stress

D. DNA damage

1506. All of the following are possible environment estrogen receptor agonists except _____.

A. methoxychlor

B. DDT

C. bromobenzene

D. bisphenol A

1507. All of the following are true of the aryl hydrocarbon receptor except _____.

A. Some very potent binders are poorly metabolized.

B. No known drugs or endogenous chemicals activate this receptor.

C. It is a ligand-binding cytosolic receptor.

D. Genes upregulated by the receptor include specific P450s.

1508. An important organ in fish for the assessment of toxicologic effects is _____.

A. gill
B. eye
C. fin
D. barbels

1509. Studies done on zebrafish have suggested that observed developmental toxicity is due to stimulation of the _____.

A. estrogen receptor
B. constitutive androstane receptor
C. pregnane X receptor
D. aryl hydrocarbon receptor

1510. The most common group of chemicals implicated in causing liver cancers in fish are _____.

A. hormonal disruptors
B. heavy metals
C. polyaromatic hydrocarbons
D. carbonate pesticides

1511. The microgram mass of a toxin in an organism per kilogram of lipid divided by the microgram mass of the toxin in a sediment per kilogram of carbon is called _____.

A. bioconcentration factor
B. sediment bioavailability
C. food chain ratio
D. biota sediment accumulation factor

CHAPTER 25 ANSWERS (REFERENCES)

1476. D (I)
1477. B (I)
1478. C (I)
1479. B (I)
1480. C (II)
1481. A (II)
1482. D (II)
1483. C (II)
1484. A (II)
1485. B (I)
1486. A (I)
1487. D (I)
1488. C (I)
1489. C (I)
1490. D (I)
1491. D (I)
1492. C (I)
1493. B (I)
1494. A (I)
1495. C (I)
1496. B (I)
1497. A (I)
1498. A (I)
1499. A (I)
1500. A (I)
1501. D (I)
1502. B (I)
1503. C (I)
1504. D (I)
1505. A (I)
1506. C (I)
1507. B (I)
1508. A (I)
1509. D (I)
1510. C (I)
1511. D (I)

REFERENCES

CHAPTER 25

I.   R. T. DiGuilio and M. C. Newman, "Ecotoxicology," in *Casarett & Doull's Toxicology: The Basic Science of Poisons*, 7th ed., ed. C. D. Klaassen (New York: McGraw-Hill, 2008), 1157–1188.

II. M. A. Lewis, A. Fairbrother, and R. E. Menzer, "Methods in Environmental Toxicology," in *Principles and Methods of Toxicology*, 5th ed., ed. A. W. Hayes (Boca Raton: Taylor and Francis, 2008), 2113–2154.

26

AIR AND WATER POLLUTION

1512. The Clean Air Act of 1970 established _____.

   A. OHSA
   B. USEPA
   C. FDA
   D. USDA

1513. Approximately what percent of the United States' population lives in areas that are noncompliant with NAAQS?

   A. 10
   B. 20
   C. 50
   D. 90

1514. How many chemicals are listed as hazardous air pollutants (HAPs) under the Clean Air Act Amendment of 1990?

   A. 8
   B. 26
   C. 188
   D. 421

1515. In terms of excess mortality, particulate-matter air pollution is most pronounced in _____.

    A. Eastern Europe
    B. United States
    C. Latin America
    D. India

1516. All of the following are fuel additives except _____.

    A. hexachlorophene
    B. organic oxygenates
    C. methylcyclopentadienyl manganese tricarbonyl
    D. platinum compounds

1517. All of the following are common symptoms associated with sick building syndrome except _____.

    A. memory loss
    B. headaches
    C. fatigue
    D. nausea

1518. A gas that is water-soluble and can cause bronchoconstriction and mucus secretion in humans is _____.

    A. ozone
    B. nitrogen dioxide
    C. sulfur dioxide
    D. carbon monoxide

1519. Most of the irritant acid sulfates in air are neutralized by _____.

    A. sodium bicarbonate
    B. ammonia
    C. sodium hydroxide
    D. sodium carbonate

1520. Which of the following statements is true?

A. Ozone does not stimulate neutrophilic lung inflammation.
B. Inhaled sulfuric acid disturbs eicosanoid homeostasis.
C. Inhaled sulfuric acid stimulates neutrophilic lung inflammation.
D. The primary concern with exposure to inhaled sulfuric acid is long-term disease secondary to connective tissue disturbances.

1521. The index that most correlates with the biological effects of PM is _____.

A. percent organic composition
B. percent metal composition
C. percent total inorganic composition
D. mass concentration

1522. Which of the following would likely have the lowest ratio of indoor to outdoor concentration in air?

A. carbon monoxide
B. particulate matter
C. VOCs
D. ozone

1523. A meteorological inversion is _____.

A. cold air capped over warm air
B. warm air capped over cold air
C. vertical mixing of cold air over warm air
D. vertical mixing of warm air over cold air

1524. The organ thought to be affected most by particulate-matter air pollution is _____.

A. liver
B. heart

C. brain
D. skin

1525. All of the following are considered plausible reasons to explain the biological hazards of particulate matter air pollution except _____.

A. presence of metals
B. presence of viruses
C. presence of organics
D. presence of oxidants

1526. The results of the Harvard Six Cities Study demonstrated all of the following except _____.

A. The presence of PM had a significant effect on life span.
B. Presence of acid in pollution correlated better than sulfate for causing bronchitis in children.
C. Presence of sulfate in pollution was better associated with acute mortality than acid.
D. Presence of acid in air pollution was better associated with acute mortality than sulfate.

1527. All of the following groups are more sensitive to air pollutants except _____.

A. asthmatics
B. farmers
C. elderly
D. children

1528. The air pollutant that has undergone the most significant decrease since 1973 is _____.

A. carbon monoxide
B. ozone
C. lead
D. volatile organic compounds (VOCs)

1529. Which of the following air pollutants has had the largest percentage decrease since 1993?

    A. sulfur dioxide
    B. carbon monoxide
    C. nitrogen oxide
    D. particulate matter

1530. Reducing-type air pollutants have historically been associated with _____.

    A. coal-based urban centers
    B. suburban areas
    C. rural farm areas
    D. areas having less than 10 inches of annual rainfall

1531. All of the following statements are true except _____.

    A. It is estimated that over 480 million people worldwide are exposed to potentially harmful levels of ozone.
    B. People in most industrialized countries spend more than 80 % of their time indoors.
    C. Children are more likely to be exposed to higher levels of outdoor air pollutants compared to adults.
    D. Historically, oxidant-type air pollution was more likely to occur during winter months.

1532. Ultrafine particles are defined as _____.

    A. $< 0.001 \mu m$
    B. $< 0.01 \mu m$
    C. $< 0.1 \mu m$
    D. $< 2.5 \mu m$

1533. All of the following statements are true regarding diesel emissions except _____.

    A. Particulate emissions are largely ultrafine.
    B. Diesel exhaust induces inflammation in human airway cells.

C. Ozone enhances the toxicity of diesel particles alone.
D. Unlike gasoline, diesel exhaust does not contain a significant amount of sulfur dioxide, nitrogen dioxide, and VOCs.

1534. Lung cancer has been caused in rats by overload with all of the following except _____.

A. humidified air
B. toner dust
C. talc
D. diesel emissions

1535. The fact that coal miners do not seem to have a higher risk of lung cancer if they are not smokers supports the concept that _____.

A. Overload lung cancer may not be relevant to humans.
B. Human lungs have different P450s compared to a rat's.
C. Human lungs have different blood flow from rat lungs.
D. all of the above

1536. All of the following are components of photochemical air pollution except _____.

A. ozone
B. nitric oxides
C. argon
D. peroxyacetyl nitrates

1537. Ozone reacts with unsaturated fatty acids in the lung to form all of the following except _____.

A. hydroxyhydroperoxides
B. aldehydes
C. alkanes
D. ozonides

1538. All of the following are true of ozone except _____.

    A. It can decrease the incidence of infection in animals exposed to aerosols containing infectious agents.
    B. Toxicity may vary according to genetics.
    C. It can induce tolerance to itself.
    D. Some studies have shown that antioxidant supplements can protect against ozone's toxic effects.

1539. All of the following are true of nitrogen dioxide except _____.

    A. Farmers can be exposed to near-lethal levels.
    B. It can cause pulmonary edema.
    C. It is a more potent irritant than ozone.
    D. It is a deep lung irritant.

1540. Nitrogen dioxide is associated with all of the following except _____.

    A. indoor kerosene heaters
    B. sidestream tobacco smoke
    C. fresh silage
    D. blue-green algae

1541. All of the following are true of carbon monoxide except _____.

    A. It is highly water-soluble.
    B. It is not a deep lung irritant.
    C. It can decrease coronary sinus $pO2$ in patients with coronary artery disease.
    D. The normal concentration of carboxyhemoglobin in nonsmokers is 0.5 %.

1542. A genetic variation in which of the following enzymes has been associated with an enhancement of allergic airway inflammation in people exposed to diesel exhaust particles?

    A. CYP2D6
    B. glutathione-S-transference M1

C. cyclooxygenase 2

D. glucuronyl transferase

1543. Airborne concentrators of which of the following has stopped being a major health problem in the United States?

A. sulfur dioxide

B. nitrogen dioxide

C. lead

D. ozone

1544. A compound added to gasoline to reduce wintertime carbon monoxide emissions is _____.

A. chloroform

B. methyl tert-butyl ether

C. dimethyltin

D. xylene

1545. The guinea pig is a better model than the rat for _____.

A. upper airway irritant responses

B. tissue remodeling

C. nasal tumors

D. none of the above

1546. The major air pollutant emitted in the United States is _____.

A. nitrogen dioxide

B. carbon monoxide

C. sulfur dioxide

D. ozone

1547. All of the following are potential indoor air pollution carcinogens except _____.

A. radon

B. formaldehyde

C. 1,3-butadine

D. tobacco smoke

1548. A characteristic of the sick building syndrome is _____.

A. Legionnaires' disease, accounting for up to 20 % of cases.
B. It is frequently associated with a low-grade fever.
C. Reproducibility in animals is a diagnostic criterion.
D. Specific etiology is frequently unknown.

1549. The Clean Air Act of 1970 adopted standards for air levels of all of the following except _____.

A. ozone
B. carbon monoxide
C. carbon dioxide
D. particulate matter

Matching Test

1550. biochemical oxygen demand   A. pulp and paper industry

1551. arsenic water pollution   B. cooling tower waste

1552. TCDD water pollution   C. semiconductor industry

1553. hexavalent chromium water   D. mining and mineral
      pollution   industry

1554. halohydrocarbon water   E. related to microbe levels
      pollution   in drinking water

CHAPTER 26 ANSWERS (REFERENCES)

1512. B (I)
1513. C (I)
1514. C (I)
1515. D (I)
1516. A (I)
1517. A (I)
1518. C (I)
1519. B (I)
1520. B (I)
1521. D (I)
1522. D (I)
1523. A (I)
1524. B (I)
1525. B (I)
1526. D (I)
1527. B (I)
1528. C (I)
1529. A (I)
1530. A (I)
1531. D (I)
1532. C (I)
1533. D (I)
1534. A (II)
1535. A (II)
1536. C (I)
1537. C (I)
1538. A (I)
1539. C (I)
1540. D (I)
1541. A (I)
1542. B (III)
1543. C (III)
1544. B (I)
1545. A (I)
1546. B (I)
1547. C (I)

1548. D (I)
1549. C (I)
1550. E (IV)
1551. D (IV)
1552. A (IV)
1553. B (IV)
1554. C (IV)

REFERENCES

CHAPTER 26

I. C. L. Costa CL, "Air Pollution," in *Casarett & Doull's Toxicology: The Basic Science of Poisons*, 7th ed., ed. C. D. Klaassen (New York: McGraw-Hill, 2008), 1119–1156.

II. R. Valentine and G. L. Kennedy, "Inhalation Toxicology," in *Principles and Methods of Toxicology*, 5th ed., ed. A. W. Hayes (Boca Raton: Taylor and Francis, 2008), 1407–1464.

II. J. R. Balmes, "Outdoor Air Pollution," in *Current Occupational and Environmental Medicine*, 4th ed., ed. J. Landou (New York: McGraw-Hill, 2007), 702–709

III. D. T. Teitebaum and T. K. Joshi, "Water Pollution," in *Current Occupational and Environmental Medicine*, 4th ed., ed. J. Landou (New York: McGraw-Hill, 2007), 730–748.

27

FOOD TOXICOLOGY

1555. The major concern for food safety worldwide is _____.

    A. unregulated food additives
    B. geographic variation in soil
    C. microbial contamination
    D. radiation of food

1556. The basic presumption of the United States regarding food is
_____.

    A. All food without additives or contaminants is safe.
    B. Food from plant sources is safe.
    C. Food must be periodically tested for safety.
    D. Food additives before 1980 are safe.

1557. Tripalmitin has been shown to _____.

    A. increase gastric pH
    B. increase intestinal transit time
    C. decrease gastric emptying
    D. increase lymph flow

1558. GRAS substances added to food _____.

    A. are all food colors
    B. can be certified based on experience before 1958

C. can include pesticides

D. must have an upper limit

1559. Unavoidable contaminants to food _____.

A. have tolerance limits

B. include pesticide residues

C. include aflatoxins

D. all of the above

1560. Which of the following is true for color food additives?

A. They all contain the prefix FD and C.

B. They must come from plants.

C. They interact with antihypertensive medication.

D. They are not eligible for GRAS status.

1561. The principal reason for the low toxicity of aromatic amine color food additives is _____.

A. Sulfonation to highly polar, poorly absorbable molecules.

B. They decompose in the acid environment of the stomach.

C. They are substrates for intestinal efflux transporters.

D. The parent compounds are incapable of forming electrophiles.

1562. Caramel is considered _____.

A. a food color additive that is exempt from certification

B. a food color additive that requires individual-batch chemical analysis

C. a food color adjunct

D. a flavor enhancer

1563. Butylated hydroxyanisole (BHA) is considered ____.

A. an emulsifier

B. a buffering agent

C. a preservative

D. a dough strengthener

1564. All of the following are nonnutritive sweeteners except _____.

A. acesulfame
B. aspartame
C. saccharin
D. gum arabic

1565. Sodium benzoate is used in food as _____.

A. a processing aid
B. a firming agent
C. an antimicrobial agent
D. a drying agent

1566. All of the following are true of food color additives except _____.

A. Fifty percent of United States' food contains a color additive.
B. The average daily intake is about 15 mg.
C. The maximum daily intake is about 54 mg.
D. Beverages contain a large quantity.

1567. The NOAEL divided by 100 for a food additive is a starting point for _____.

A. chronic animal-toxicity studies
B. GRAS tolerance limits
C. estimated daily intake (EDI)
D. acceptable daily intake (ADI)

1568. A food additive containing an α, β-unsaturated carbonyl function would be most likely assigned to structure category _____.

A. A
B. B
C. C
D. D

1569. In utero testing of food additives began because of problems with _____.

A. BHA
B. saccharin
C. FD & C Blue No. 1
D. papain

1570. Indirect food additives _____.

A. are produced from microbial contamination of food
B. enter food from surfaces that contact food
C. are chemicals that result from the transformation of food substances by the cooking process
D. all of the above

1571. Significant migration of indirect food additives in extraction studies is defined as _____.

A. 0.1to 1 ppb
B. 1 to 10 ppb
C. 10 to 50 ppb
D. 50 to 1000 ppb

1572. All of the following are considered GRAS except _____.

A. patulin
B. helium
C. acetic acid
D. aluminum calcium silicate

1573. All of the following are true of GRAS status except _____.

A. It is based on safety as assessed by common knowledge throughout the scientific community.
B. It can be based on experiences with common use in food before January 1, 1958.
C. GRAS substances are still subject to the Delaney Clause.
D. New data can change the GRAS status of a substance.

1574. Which of the following is true regarding dietary supplements?

    A. They are considered food additives.
    B. They are considered drugs.
    C. The daily recommended intake is not stated on the product label.
    D. There is an implied assumption of some risk on the part of the consumer.

1575. The Delaney Clause applies to all of the following except _____.

    A. unavoidable contaminants
    B. food additives
    C. color additives
    D. animal drugs

1576. The DES proviso of the Delaney Clause _____.

    A. restricts endocrine disrupters in animal feed
    B. allow for carcinogens in animal feed if there is no residue in the edible tissue
    C. allows for DES in animal feed at a level below the NOAEL for feminizing a male fetus
    D. none of the above

1577. All of the following have been banned food additives because of the Delaney Clause except _____.

    A. Flectol H
    B. safrole
    C. xylitol
    D. thiourea

1578. The reasoning behind why a chemical like sorbitol, which is listed as a carcinogen in some data bases, is still listed by the FDA as a food additive is _____.

    A. only animal and no human evidence for carcinogenicity.
    B. it was found to be safe prior to 1958

C. threshold-dose response has been confirmed and is above average daily intake.

D. cancer is caused by secondary carcinogenesis.

1579. Which of the following drug–food interaction pairs is incorrect?

A. cyclosporin–grapefruit juice
B. MAO inhibitors–cheese
C. vitamin C–carrots
D. tetracycline-milk

1580. All of the following food–allergic protein pairs is correct except?

A. egg whites–ovomucoid
B. peanuts–Ara h II
C. egg yolks–livetin
D. cow's milk–gluten

1581. All of the following are true of food idiosyncrasy except _____.

A. It may have a genetic basis.
B. Lactose intolerance is an example.
C. Peanut allergy is not an example.
D. Immune mechanisms are involved.

1582. A reaction to tuna or mackerel that appears like an allergic reaction would most likely be classified as _____.

A. idiosyncratic
B. anaphylactoid
C. food poisoning
D. food anaphylaxis

1583. Food anaphylaxis is most common with _____.

A. peas
B. soybeans
C. peanuts

D. lentils

1584. Hemolysis has been associated with ingestion of _____.

A. fava beans
B. chocolate
C. asparagus
D. rice

1585. Red urine that can mimic hematuria can be caused by _____.

A. red wine
B. red beets
C. red cabbage
D. red onions

1586. In sensitive individuals exposed to sulfites, a deficiency of sulfite oxidase can produce _____.

A. hypertension
B. diarrhea
C. bronchospasm
D. mental confusion

1587. All of the following food–CYP450 enzyme interaction pairs are correct except _____.

A. cheese-2D6
B. watercress-2E1
C. grapefruit juice–3A4
D. charred meat–1A2

1588. All of the following food–metabolic interaction pairs are correct except _____.

A. cabbage-goiter
B. licorice-hypertension
C. polar bear liver–vitamin A toxicity
D. cycad flour–toxic epidermal necrolysis

1589. Isothiocyanates and thiocyanates are present the least in
_____.

    A. mustard
    B. broccoli
    C. horseradish
    D. potato

1590. All of the following mycotoxin-effect pairs are correct except
_____.

    A. trichothecenes–hematopoetic toxicity
    B. fumonisins–cardiac beriberi
    C. ochratoxin-nephropathy
    D. zearalenones–estrogenic effects

1591. Solanine and chaconine are produced in _____.

    A. broccoli
    B. cabbage
    C. potato
    D. corn

1592 Trans fat has been found to _____.

    A. increase blood glucose
    B. raise HDL cholesterol
    C. raise LDL cholesterol
    D. raise blood pressure

1593. The toxin in amnesic shellfish poisoning resembles _____.

    A. glycine
    B. dopamine
    C. acetylcholine
    D. glutamine

1594. All of the following are true regarding tetrodotoxin except _____.

    A. It can be present in puffer fish, frogs, and octopus.
    B. It works by increasing inward sodium ion movement in the neuron.
    C. It is associated with the presence of certain bacteria.
    D. It is stable in boiling water.

1595. Iodine excess could result from consuming large amounts of _____.

    A. cod
    B. kelp
    C. goat's milk
    D. soybeans

1596. In the United States, the regulation of pesticide residues is under the jurisdiction of the _____.

    A. EPA
    B. FDA
    C. OHSA
    D. NAS

1597. The highest amount of dietary arsenic comes from the consumption of _____.

    A. red meat
    B. poultry
    C. seafood
    D. cow's milk

1598. Well water can be a significant source of _____.

    A. perchlorate
    B. sulfite
    C. thiocyanate
    D. nitrate

1599. All of the following are true regarding N-nitrosoproline except _____.

    A. It is a definite human carcinogen.
    B. It is a nitrosoamine.
    C. It is excreted unchanged in the urine.
    D. It is common in humans.

1600. The major complication of Half disease is _____.

    A. rhabdomyolysis
    B. liver failure
    C. congestive heart failure
    D. pulmonary fibrosis

1601. All of the following statements are true regarding botulinum toxin except _____.

    A. It is heat resistant to 150 °C.
    B. It is a zinc metalloprotein.
    C. The lethal dose is approximately 1 nanogram.
    D. It is structurally similar to tetanus toxin.

1602. A common feature of toxins produced by C. perfringens, E.coli, and B.cereus is _____.

    A. respiratory paralysis
    B. clotting abnormalities
    C. diarrheal illness
    D. toxic shock syndrome

1603. Bovine spongiform encephalopathy is caused by a _____.

    A. protozoa
    B. bacteria
    C. virus
    D. prion

1604. Heterocyclic amines and acrylamide are food contaminants which _____.

    A. are produced by microorganisms
    B. are produced by the process of cooking
    C. are considered GRAS
    D. are residues from animal feeds

1605. The concept of "de minimis" as applied to food safety means _____.

    A. Find the smallest harmful dose
    B. Only food colors at 1/100 of the NOAEL can be used.
    C. Pesticide residues can be present at the ADI.
    D. The risk is so small it is of no concern.

Matching Test

1606. *E. coli*   A. mahimahi

1607. ciguatera poisoning   B. GRAS substance

1608. endotoxin   C. gram-negative bacterial toxin

1609. emetic toxin   D. enzyme

1610. fluoride   E. apple products

1611. scombroid poisoning   F. beets

1612. iron oxide   G. *B. cereus*

1613. rennet   H. dinoflagellates

1614. patulin   I. contaminant in hamburger meat, raw vegetables

1615. high nitrates   J. osteosclerosis

CHAPTER 27 ANSWERS (REFERENCES)

1555.	C (I)	1591.	C (I)
1556.	A (I)	1592.	C (I)
1557.	D (I)	1593.	D (I)
1558.	B (I)	1594.	B (I)
1559.	D (I)	1595.	B (I)
1560.	D (I)	1596.	A (I)
1561.	A (I)	1597.	C (I)
1562.	A (I)	1598.	D (I)
1563.	C (I)	1599.	A (I)
1564.	D (I)	1600.	A (I)
1565.	C (I)	1601.	A (I)
1566.	A (I)	1602.	C (I)
1567.	D (I)	1603.	D (I)
1568.	C (I)	1604.	B (I)
1569.	B (I)	1605.	D (I)
1570.	B (I)	1606.	I (I)
1571.	D (I)	1607.	H (I)
1572.	A (I)	1608.	C (I)
1573.	C (I)	1609.	G (I)
1574.	D (I)	1610.	J (I)
1575.	A (I)	1611.	A (I)
1576.	B (I)	1612.	B (I)
1577.	C (I)	1613.	D (I)
1578.	D (I)	1614.	E (I)
1579.	C (I)	1615.	F (I)
1580.	D (I)		
1581.	D (I)		
1582.	B (I)		
1583.	C (I)		
1584.	A (I)		
1585.	B (I)		
1586.	C (I)		
1587.	A (I)		
1588.	D (I)		
1589.	D (I)		
1590.	B (I)		

REFERENCES

CHAPTER 27

I.   F. N. Kotsonis and G. A. Burdock, "Food Toxicology," in *Casarett & Doull's Toxicology: The Basic Science of Poisons*, 7th ed., ed. C. D. Klaassen (New York: McGraw-Hill, 2008), 1191–1237.

28

OCCUPATIONAL TOXICOLOGY

1616. Dose in an occupational setting is a function of _____.

    A. exposure concentration
    B. exposure frequency
    C. exposure duration
    D. all of the above

1617. All of the following are determinants of an inhalation exposure except _____.

    A. tidal volume
    B. respiratory rate
    C. blood pressure
    D. airborne concentration

1618. All of the following are determinants of a skin exposure except _____.

    A. region of skin exposed
    B. respiratory rate
    C. surface area exposed
    D. preexisting skin disease

1619. An occupational exposure limit that is averaged over an 8-hour workday, 5-day workweek is

A. TLV-TWA
B. TLV-STEL
C. TLV-C
D. TLV-OEL

1620. An occupational exposure limit for a 15-minute period is _____.

A. TLV-TWA
B. TLV-STEL
C. TLV-C
D. TLV-OEL

1621. Occupational asthma is highest in _____.

A. construction workers
B. farmers
C. general merchandise stores
D. lifeguards

1622. All of the following statements are true regarding biological monitoring of exposed workers except _____.

A. It can be used to test the efficiency of personal protective equipment.
B. It is more directly related to adverse health effects than environmental monitoring.
C. It accounts for uptake by all exposure routes.
D. It is generally less expensive and less invasive than environmental monitoring.

1623. All of the following are disadvantages of biological monitoring except _____.

A. It is not useful for dermally corrosive agents.
B. It is limited to urine testing.

C. It is not useful for primary lung irritants.

D. It is not useful for assessing damage from peak effects of chemicals.

1624. Para-aminophenol is a urine biomarker for exposure to _____.

A. aniline
B. benzene
C. styrene
D. phenol

1625. Urine oxalic acid is a biomarker for exposure to _____.

A. trichloroethylene
B. ethylene glycol
C. isopropyl alcohol
D. allyl alcohol

1626. An occupational exposure limit that should never be exceeded is _____.

A. TLV-TWA
B. TLV-STEL
C. TLV-C
D. TLV-OEL

1627. Silica and asbestos are associated with _____.

A. renal carcinoma
B. asthma
C. fibrotic lung disease
D. nasal carcinoma

1628. Both coal dust and cigarette smoke are associated with _____.

A. emphysema
B. non-Hodgkin's lymphoma

C. bladder carcinoma

D. soft tissue sarcoma

1629. Carbon monoxide has been associated with _____.

A. asthma and multiple sclerosis

B. asphyxiation and Parkinson's disease

C. hypersensitivity pneumonitis and hemolysis

D. nasal polyps and peripheral neuropathy

1630. Thermophilic bacteria have been associated with _____.

A. toxic shock syndrome

B. Steven-Johnson syndrome

C. encephalitis

D. hypersensitivity pneumonitis

1631. Chronic bronchospasm after a single high-dose exposure to a chemical respiratory irritant is termed _____.

A. occupational asthma

B. hypersensitivity pneumonitis

C. reactive airway dysfunction syndrome (RADS)

D. allergic alveolitis

1632. A chemical in epoxy resins associated with pulmonary hemorrhage-anemia syndrome in workers is _____.

A. sodium sulfite

B. trimellitic anhydride

C. propylene glycol

D. butter yellow

1633. An aerosol of liquid particles is called _____.

A. mist

B. fume

C. gas

D. dust

1634. All of the following are considered simple asphyxiants except
_____.

A. acetylene
B. oxygen
C. hydrogen
D. nitrogen

1635. All of the following are considered toxic asphyxiants except
_____.

A. carbon monoxide
B. hydrogen cyanide
C. hydrogen sulfide
D. nitrous oxide

1636. Dust from the earth's crust is mostly deposited in _____.

A. upper airways
B. medium airways
C. lower airways
D. pulmonary artery

1637. All of the following are common components of smoke from
industrial fires except _____.

A. carbon monoxide
B. particulate matter
C. styrene
D. formaldehyde

1638. A problem with collecting air samples in evacuated containers
is _____.

A. Samples can react or degrade in a short period
B. Temperature differences between collection location and
analysis location can interfere with results.

C. Heavier gases cannot be completely removed from the container.

D. all of the above

1639. All of the following are media for the collection of gases and vapors for environmental testing except _____.

A. charcoal
B. silica gel
C. calcium carbonate
D. gas chromatography column-packing material

1640. A useful device to detect the pressure of a gas or vapor above a threshold toxic level without requiring the services of a person with specialized training is _____.

A. gas chromatograph
B. liquid chromatograph
C. liquid media collector
D. color-changing badge

Matching Test

1641. chlorine

1642. phosgene

1643. ozone

1644. ethylene oxide

1645. formaldehyde

1646. nitrogen dioxide

1647. ammonia

1648. arsine

1649. methyl bromide

1650. chloroacetophenone

1651. zinc chloride

1652. hydrogen sulfide

1653. methane

1654. argon

1655. hydrofluoric acid

1656. carbon monoxide

1657. carbon dioxide

A. microelectronics industry

B. furniture manufacturers

C. glass etching

D. beer and wine fermentation

E. gas sterilizing systems

F. water treatment workers

G. arc welders and printers

H. simple asphyxiant in coal mines

I. inert gas simple asphyxiant

J. sewage and manure workers

K. tear gas

L. fertilizer manufacturing

M. agricultural workers

N. pesticide manufacturing, welding

O. fumigant applicators

P. group symptoms confused with food poisoning

Q. smoke bombs

CHAPTER 28 ANSWERS (REFERENCES)

1616.	D (I)	1652.	J (III)
1617.	C (I)	1653.	H (III)
1618.	B (I)	1654.	I (III)
1619.	A (I)	1655.	C (V)
1620.	B (I)	1656.	P (III)
1621.	C (I)	1657.	D (III)
1622.	D (I)		
1623.	B (I)		
1624.	A (I)		
1625.	B (I)		
1626.	C (I)		
1627.	C (I)		
1628.	A (I)		
1629.	B (I)		
1630.	D (I)		
1631.	C (I)		
1632.	B (II)		
1633.	A (III)		
1634.	B (III)		
1635.	D (III)		
1636.	A (II)		
1637.	C (III)		
1638.	A (IV)		
1639.	C (IV)		
1640.	D (IV)		
1641.	F (III)		
1642.	N (III)		
1643.	G (III)		
1644.	E (III)		
1645.	B (III)		
1646.	M (III)		
1647.	L (III)		
1648.	A (III)		
1649.	O (III)		
1650.	K (III)		
1651.	Q (III)		

REFERENCES

CHAPTER 28

I. P. S. Thorne, "Occupational Toxicology," in *Casarett & Doull's Toxicology: The Basic Science of Poisons*, 7th ed., ed. C. D. Klaassen (New York: McGraw-Hill, 2008), 1273–1292.

II. J. R. Balmes, "Occupational Lung Diseases," in *Current Occupational and Environmental Medicine*, 4th ed., ed. J. Landou (New York: McGraw-Hill, 2007), 310–333.

III. W. G. Kuschner and P. D. Blanc, "Gases and Other Airborne Toxicants," in *Current Occupational and Environmental Medicine*, 4th ed., ed. J. Landou (New York: McGraw-Hill, 2007), 515–531.

IV. D. P. Fowler, "Industrial (Occupational) Hygiene," in *Current Occupational and Environmental Medicine*, 4th ed., ed. J. Landou (New York: McGraw-Hill, 2007), 613–628.

V. R. J. Harrison, "Chemicals," in *Current Occupational and Environmental Medicine*, 4th ed., J. Landou (New York: McGraw-Hill, 2007), 439–480.

29

ANALYTICAL TOXICOLOGY

1658. The largest group of substances that must be considered by analytical toxicologists is/are_____.

  A. nonvolatile organic substances
  B. metals
  C. gases
  D. volatile substances

1659. If a human tissue sample in question is made basic and extracted with organic solvent and then the nonorganic phase is acidified and extracted again with organic solvent, the final organic extract will contain mostly _____.

  A. basic drugs
  B. neutral drugs
  C. acidic drugs
  D. volatiles

1660. Venoms usually need to be measured by a combination of monoclonal antibodies and _____.

  A. gas chromatography
  B. infrared spectroscopy
  C. liquid chromatography
  D. immunoassay

1661. Analytic toxicology measurements are least useful in_____.

A. establishing bioavailability of a poorly absorbed drug
B. assessing pharmacodynamic drug interactions
C. identifying contaminants in a drug mixture
D. assessing pharmacokinetic drug interactions

1662. In order for an analytic toxicology result to be entered into legal proceedings, there usually must be _____.

A. chain of custody
B. 3 repeat analyses
C. blood results, not tissue or urine
D. analysis by a board-certified forensic toxicologist

1663. The precision of an analytic toxicology result is related to _____.

A. location value falls on standard curve
B. accuracy of value on repeat measurements
C. whether dilution was necessary
D. accuracy of value in blood compared to tissue

1664. Identification of anhydroecgonine methyl ester along with cocaine metabolites in the urine is an indicator that _____.

A. Cocaine was adulterated with PCP.
B. Cocaine was administered orally.
C. Cocaine was smoked.
D. Cocaine was taken with ethyl alcohol.

1665. The least useful specimen for quantitative toxicologic analysis is _____.

A. blood
B. liver
C. urine
D. vitreous human

1666. By identifying the presence of certain impurities in biological samples obtained after consumption of an illicitly produced drug, analytic toxicologists may be able to _____.

   A. more accurately predict the time of ingestion
   B. more accurately predict the mode of ingestion
   C. more accurately predict the likelihood of a drug interaction
   D. possibly identify the source of the illicit material

1667. The classic Mickey Finn of the nineteenth century was a mixture of ethyl alcohol and _____.

   A. isopropyl alcohol
   B. chloral hydrate
   C. butalbital
   D. meprobamate

1668. A child who is intentionally poisoned by parents to repeatedly appear ill is part of the syndrome known as _____.

   A. Munchausen syndrome
   B. Munchausen syndrome by proxy
   C. borderline personality syndrome
   D. DSM IV syndrome

1669. The most common drug/drug class found in victims of sexual assault is _____.

   A. marijuana
   B. ethyl alcohol
   C. benzodiazepines
   D. opiates

1670. Analysis of how much hair will provide an approximate monthly pattern of arsenic exposure?

   A. 1 mm
   B. 5 mm

C. 12 mm
D. 25 mm

1671. All of the following tests can help detect adulteration of a urine specimen for forensic testing except _____.

A. pH
B. creatinine
C. specific gravity
D. pressure of WBCs

1672. In order to distinguish heroin use from poppy seed ingestion, analysis should be performed for the presence of _____.

A. 6-monacetylmorphine
B. morphine glucuronide
C. codeine
D. hydromorphone

1673. All of the following are commonly used to adulterate urine for drug testing purposes except _____.

A. bleach
B. baking soda
C. glutaraldehyde
D. methylene blue

1674. Use of a Vicks inhaler may result in a false positive urinary drug screen for _____.

A. opiates
B. PCP
C. D-methamphetamine
D. L-methamphetamine

1675. A rapid quantitative determination of serum concentrations of all of the following drugs is required in an overdose setting except _____.

A. acetaminophen
B. ethanol
C. ibuprofen
D. ethylene glycol

1676. A commonly used term to denote the serum level of a drug that should be immediately reported to the treating physician is _____.

A. panic level
B. lethal level
C. toxic level
D. subtherapeutic level

1677. Traditionally, therapeutic drug monitoring has been performed on all of the following drug classes except _____.

A. antimicrobials
B. antihypertensives
C. anticonvulsants
D. antiarrhythmins

1678. In usual cases, toxicologic analysis of dead bodies has involved the use of all of the following except _____.

A. maggots
B. hair
C. clothing
D. bones

1679. Interference with toxicologic analysis will least likely result from contaminants present in _____.

A. specimen containers
B. air

C. lids

D. stoppers

1680. When analyzing a specimen where extraction efficiency is highly variable, one can use the method of _____.

A. standard additions

B. least squares

C. standard curves

D. internal standards

1681. Which of the following would be expected to have the highest degree of postmortem redistribution?

A. mercuric ion

B. ethanol

C. paraquat

D. imipramine

1682. Which of the following is true of a urine drug screen?

A. Chain of custody is not required for forensic evidence.

B. Over 50 drug classes can be rapidly screened.

C. There is a poor correlation between levels and clinical effects.

D. They are commonly run by HPLC.

Matching Test

1683. spot test

1684. HPLC

1685. TLC

1686. GC

1687. GC/MS

1688. immunoassay

1689. spectrochemical

1690. LC/MS/MS

A. nonquantitative, can screen many drugs/metabolites at one time

B. Noncompetitive and competitive types exist.

C. Detector bombards molecules with electron stream.

D. simplest and fastest test

E. typically uses reverse phase conditions

F. commonly uses flame ionization detector

G. detector adds or removes protons

H. quantitative test relying on light absorption

CHAPTER 29 ANSWERS (REFERENCES)

1658. A (I)
1659. C (I)
1660. D (I)
1661. B (I)
1662. A (I)
1663. B (I)
1664. C (I)
1665. C (I)
1666. D (I)
1667. B (I)
1668. B (I)
1669. B (I)
1670. C (I)
1671. D (I)
1672. A (I)
1673. D (I)
1674. C (I)
1675. C (I)
1676. A (I)
1677. B (I)
1678. C (I)
1679. B (I)
1680. A (I)
1681. D (I)
1682. C (I)
1683. D (II)
1684. E (II)
1685. A (II)
1686. F (II)
1687. C (II)
1688. B (II)
1689. H (II)
1690. G (II)

REFERENCES

CHAPTER 29

I. A. Poklis, "Analytic/Forensic Toxicology," in *Casarett & Doull's Toxicology: The Basic Science of Poisons*, 7th ed., ed. C. D. Klaassen (New York: McGraw-Hill, 2008), 1237–1256.

II. P. M. Rainey, "Laboratory Principles," in *Goldfrank's Toxicologic Emergencies*, 9th ed., ed. L. S. Nelson et al. (New York: McGraw-Hill, 2011), 70–89.

30

DRUG ABUSE TOXICOLOGY

1691. An estimation of the amount of cocaine use in a community could best come from _____.

A. hospital admissions
B. police arrests
C. concentration of metabolites in water supply
D. interviews

1692. In 2003, the leading 2 illicit drugs causing death reported to the Drug Abuse Warning Network (DAWN) were _____.

A. heroin and cocaine
B. methadone and fentanyl
C. methamphetamine and hydrocodone
D. cocaine and oxycodone

1693. The ratio of cocaine to benzoylecgoninc in a postmortem brain specimen can best be an indicator of _____.

A. rate of hepatic drug metabolism
B. time of ingestion
C. cause of death
D. source of drug

1694. The predominant cocaine analyte measured in human hair is _____.

    A. cocaine
    B. coacaethylene
    C. norcaine
    D. benzoylecgonine

1695. All of the following are true regarding cocaine except _____.

    A. Tolerance to its effects can develop.
    B. Myocardial fibrosis can occur in chronic users.
    C. There can be postmortem redistribution.
    D. There is a good correlation between postmortem levels and cause of death.

1696. All of the following plants produce chemicals that have a stimulant effect except _____.

    A. oleander
    B. khat
    C. ephedra
    D. absinthe

1697. All of the following are true regarding methamphetame except _____.

    A. It is N-demethylated to amphetamine.
    B. At low doses, it impairs psychomotor performance.
    C. The urine immunologic screening test is considered positive at 1,000 mg/mL or greater.
    D. Selegiline can be converted in vivo to methamphetamine.

1698. In the presence of ethanol, cocaine will be metabolized to _____.

    A. norcocaine
    B. methylecgonine
    C. benzoylecgonine
    D. cocaethylene

1699. The major pyrolysis product of cocaine is _____.

    A. norcocaine
    B. methylecgonine
    C. anhydroecgonine methyl ester
    D. cocaethylene

1700. Cocaine is primarily metabolized by _____.

    A. CYP450 2B6
    B. glucuronidation
    C. esterases
    D. acetylation

1701. The l isomer of methamphetamine is commercially available as _____.

    A. pseudoephedrine
    B. phenylephrine
    C. Vicks decongestant
    D. phenylpropanolamine

1702. A marker for smoked methamphetamine is _____.

    A. norephedrine
    B. trans-phenylpropene
    C. O-hydroxynorphedrine
    D. P-hydroxymethamphetamine

1703. The urinary excretion of methamphetamine can be decreased by _____.

    A. phenobarbital
    B. basic urine
    C. acidic urine
    D. ammonium chloride

1704. Eighty percent of methylphenidate is excreted in the urine as
_____.

A. unchanged drug
B. ethylphenidate
C. ritalinic acid
D. amphetamine

1705. Methylphenidate differs from cocaine and amphetamine in that
_____.

A. It blocks the dopamine transporter.
B. It blocks the norepinephrine transporter.
C. It has a low affinity for the 5HT transporter.
D. It has a higher potential for abuse.

1706. GHB has increasingly been used as an agent to _____.

A. induce anesthesia
B. treat status epilepticus
C. facilitate sexual assault
D. counteract cocaine-induced delirium

1707. All of the following are true regarding dextromethorphan
except _____.

A. It has been associated with the serotonin syndrome.
B. It is highly first passed.
C. It is metabolized by CYP 2D6.
D. It is a racemic mixture.

1708. All of the following are considered benzodiazepines except
_____.

A. oxazepam
B. eszopiclone
C. chlordiazepoxide
D. clorazepate

1709. All of the following could be metabolized to oxazepam except
_____.

A. lorazepam
B. temazepam
C. diazepam
D. prazepam

1710. All of the following are true regarding benzodiazepines except
_____.

A. Withdrawal convulsions can occur.
B. Overdose of benzodiazepines alone rarely cause death.
C. Lorazepam and oxazepam do not undergo CYP450-mediated biotransformation.
D. Ibuprofen can cause a false positive result on urine screen tests.

1711. All of the following are true of normeperidine except _____.

A. It strongly binds to mu opioid receptors.
B. More is formed after oral meperidine administration than through intravenous administration
C. It causes serotonin excess in the CNS.
D. It is responsible for possible precipitation of the serotonin syndrome when meperidine is given concurrently with a MAO inhibitor.

1712. All of the following are metabolites of oxycodone except _____.

A. codeine
B. oxymorphone
C. noroxycodone
D. oxycodone glucuronide

1713. An opiate not metabolized by the P450 system is _____.

A. buprenorphine
B. fentanyl

C. oxymorphone

D. propoxyphene

1714. Propoxyphene is a derivative of _____.

A. meperidine

B. methadone

C. fentanyl

D. morphine

1715. The cardiac toxicity of propoxyphene results from _____.

A. dextropropoxyphene

B. levopropoxyphene

C. EDDP

D. norpropoxyphene

1716. The mechanism of action of phencyclidine is _____.

A. agonist at the glycine receptor

B. noncompetitive antagonist at glutamate-NMDA receptor

C. blockade of dopamine release

D. stimulation of central acetylcholine release

1717. Blood levels of phencyclidine _____.

A. strongly correlate with psychedelic effects

B. are present only for minutes before being converted to an active metabolite

C. could be present from phencyclidine use weeks before the level was drawn

D. are approximately ten times higher than brain levels

1718. All of the following are true of phencyclidine except _____.

A. It is classified as a dissociative anesthetic.

B. It can be snorted, smoke, injected, or swallowed.

C. Glucuronide metabolites are excreted in the urine.

D. Alkalinization of the urine enhances its elimination.

1719. The reason that ketamine is used for induction of anesthesia in trauma victims is that ketamine causes _____.

    A. an increase in blood pressure
    B. a blockade of the vomiting center
    C. a shortening of the QT interval
    D. a stimulation of respiration

1720. Postmortem tissue concentrates of GHB have little scientific meaning because _____.

    A. They could be present from use months before.
    B. There is a tenfold to hundredfold postmortem redistribution.
    C. The conjugated metabolites are rapidly converted back into the parent.
    D. It forms in the blood as a postmortem artifact.

1721. All of the following are true of fentanyl except _____.

    A. Sufentanil is the principal metabolite.
    B. Routine urine drug screening for drugs with an opiate nucleus will not detect it.
    C. When fentanyl patches are used to relieve chronic pain, little drug appears in the systemic circulation for the first 2 hours.
    D. Norfentanyl may appear in the urine of surgical patients for greater than 48 hours.

1722. All of the following are true of hydrocodone except _____.

    A. An intravenous form is not commercially available.
    B. It is a metabolite of codeine.
    C. It has a terminal half-life of around 4 hours.
    D. It is a mu receptor partial agonist/antagonist.

1723. All of the following are true of hydropmorphone except
_____.

A. It is more potent than morphine.
B. It is a metabolite of morphine.
C. It has a terminal half-life of 8 hours.
D. Hydromorphone-3-glucuronide is a metabolite.

1724. All of the following statements are true except _____.

A. Buprenorphine is more expensive than methadone.
B. L-LAAM was taken off the market because of QT prolongation.
C. Heroin patients receiving methadone maintenance may have improved immune function.
D. Both d and l isomers of methadone have equal potency at the mu receptor.

1725. The main metabolite of methadone is _____.

A. L-LAAM
B. EDDP
C. N-desethyl methadone
D. O-desmethyl methadone

1726. All of the following are true regarding buprenorphine except
_____.

A. It can interact with HIV medication.
B. Death rates with buprenorphine maintenance are higher than with methadone.
C. It is more potent than morphine.
D. It is classified as a partial opioid agonist.

1727. The conversion of codeine to morphine is mediated by _____.

A. CYP2E1
B. CYP3A6

    C. CYP2D6

    D. CYPIA2

1728. All of the following are possible metabolites of codeine except
_____.

    A. codeine-6-glucuronide

    B. norcodeine

    C. hydrocodone

    D. 6 acetylmorphine

1729. The least common route of fentanyl administration is _____.

    A. intramuscular

    B. transdermal

    C. intravenous

    D. transmucosal

1730. For approximately how many hours following removal of
fentanyl patch is drug still released into the systemic circulation?

    A. 1

    B. 4

    C. 12

    D. 24

1731. A level of 6 acetylmorphine in urine above the cutoff means
_____.

    A. Heroin was definitely ingested.

    B. Heroin or morphine could have been ingested.

    C. Heroin or codeine could have been ingested.

    D. Heroin or oxymorphone could have been ingested.

1732. The presence of codeine in the urine of a heroin user most
likely means _____.

    A. It was metabolized from morphine.

    B. It was a contaminant of the heroin.

C. It was deliberately co-injected with heroin.

D. It results from morphine causing a false positive result on the codeine assay.

1733. Which of the following drugs when ingested would produce a positive morphine test result on a urine drug screen ?

A. codeine
B. fentanyl
C. methadone
D. meperidine

1734. All of the following could be metabolized eventually to hydromorphone except _____.

A. codeine
B. heroin
C. morphine
D. oxycodone

1735. Morphine glucuronides are eventual metabolites of all of the following except _____.

A. morphine
B. heroin
C. hydrocodone
D. codeine

1736. Codeine can be metabolized to all of the following except _____.

A. oxycodone
B. hydrocodone
C. norcodone
D. morphine

1737. Morphine can only be metabolized to which of the following
_____.

A. heroin
B. hydrocodone
C. normorphine
D. oxymorphone

1738. Which of the following could be metabolized to morphine?

A. buprenorphine
B. oxymorphone
C. propoxyphene
D. none of the above

1739. The drug with the shortest half-life is _____.

A. buprenorphine
B. heroin
C. propoxyphene
D. methadone

1740. The opioid with the highest retail sales numbers in 2006 was
_____.

A. codeine
B. fentanyl
C. oxycodone
D. hydrocodone

1741. A spice that can act as a hallucinogen is _____.

A. paprika
B. cumin
C. coriander
D. nutmeg

1742. All of the following are true of psilocybin except _____.

    A. It is a derivative of tryptamine.
    B. Increases in pulse and blood pressure occur before psychological effects.
    C. The symptoms produced resemble schizophrenia.
    D. Effects are mediated through the 2AR-mGIuR2 receptor complex.

1743. The mechanism of psychosis in LSD is related to its binding to which receptor?

    A. D2
    B. 5-HT3
    C. 5-HT2
    D. 5-HT4

1744. The mechanism of action of LSD is most closely related to _____.

    A. PCP
    B. ketamine
    C. mescaline
    D. methylphenidate

1745. The purported fourth opiate receptor that is no longer recognized as such is _____.

    A. mu
    B. kappa
    C. sigma
    D. delta

1746. Mescaline is derived from a _____.

    A. lichen
    B. mushroom

    C. cactus

    D. moss

1747. MDMA is classified as a/an _____.

    A. dissociative anesthetic

    B. drug for ADHD

    C. hallucinogenic amphetamine

    D. anti-Parkinson drug

1748. MDMA is an inhibitor of _____.

    A. CYP2E1

    B. CYP2D6

    C. CYPIA2

    D. glucuronyl transferase

1749. The activity of MDMA is due to the central nervous system release of _____.

    A. dopamine

    B. 5-HT

    C. norepinephrine

    D. all of the above

1750. Drugs that can increase the risk of serotonin syndrome in MDMA users include all of the following except _____.

    A. meperidine

    B. nadolol

    C. tramadol

    D. dextromethorphan

1751. A finding that could support tolerance in a deceased heroin user is _____.

    A. presence of morphine throughout the hair

    B. presence of morphine in liver

C. presence of morphine in skeletal muscle

D. a morphine to morphine-3-glucuronide ratio of 6 to 1

1752. Which of the following drugs is least likely to be part of the toxicology results in a heroin-related death?

A. fentanyl

B. alcohol

C. phencyclidine

D. benzodiazepine

1753. A recently discovered mechanism for sudden death in methadone users is _____.

A. cytokine storm

B. inhibition of the hERG potassium channel

C. pulmonary embolism

D. lowering of the seizure threshold

1754. Levels of nonprotein-bound methadone would decrease in _____.

A. liver disease

B. presence of other drugs that strongly bind to alpha-1-acid glycoprotein

C. presence of other drugs that bind strongly to albumin

D. inflammatory disorders

1755. All of the following are true of methadone except _____.

A. It is metabolized by CYP3A4 and CYP2B6.

B. Its terminal half-life is very variable.

C. The d isomer strongly binds to the opiate receptor.

D. The d isomer can cause QT prolongation.

1756. A postmortem free morphine concentration value refers to _____.

A. morphine without its conjugation metabolites

B. nonprotein-bound morphine and metabolites

C. morphine, morphine glucuronide, and normorphine

D. combined level of morphine, codeine, and 6 acetylmorphine

1757. All of the following are true regarding postmortem liver opiate levels except _____.

A. Formalin embalming does not interfere with the extraction and measurement of free morphine.

B. In a nonrefrigerated cadaver, morphine glucuronide can be converted back to morphine.

C. They can be useful in some exhumations.

D. Liver 6 acetyl morphine levels are usually higher than brain levels.

1758. Poppy seed ingestion could cause a false positive urine test for all of the following except _____.

A. morphine

B. 6 acetylmorphine

C. codeine

D. morphine-6-glucuronide

1759. A substance found in poppy seeds but not in refined heroin is ____.

A. papaverine

B. noscapine

C. thebaine

D. lidocaine

1760. In order to prove heroin ingestion, 6 acetyl morphine must be present in the urine at a concentration of at least _____.

A. 10 ng/mL

B. 100 ng/mL

C. 500 ng/mL

D. 1,000 ng/mL

1761. Endogenous opiate peptides include all of the following except
_____.

A. alfentanil
B. dynorphin
C. beta-endorphin
D. endomorphin

1762. Opiate receptors are described as having _____.

A. 3 transmembrane domains
B. 5 transmembrane domains
C. 7 transmembrane domains
D. 10 transmembrane domains

1763. All of the following are common adulterants of heroin except
_____.

A. spironolactone
B. quinine
C. caffeine
D. diphenhydramine

1764. Common diluents found in heroin include all of the following
except _____.

A. lactose
B. methamphetamine
C. starch
D. mannitol

1765. The morphine metabolite that is least pharmacologically active
is _____.

A. normorphine
B. hydromorphone
C. morphine-6-glucuronide
D. morphine-3-glucuronide

1766. A test used to detect abuse of anabolic steroids is _____.

    A. serum testosterone
    B. serum-free androgens
    C. urine T/E ratio
    D. urine for total steroids

1767. All of the following are true regarding THC except _____.

    A. It binds to two known cannabinoid receptors in humans.
    B. Blood levels of the carboxylic acid metabolite in the living can reliably predict time of ingestion.
    C. Blood levels can peak very quickly.
    D. It has a high volume of distribution.

1768. Which of the following statements is most accurate regarding postmortem measurements of THC levels in blood?

    A. They are extremely difficult to interpret with respect to time of use.
    B. THC levels are more accurate than 11-OH-THC levels.
    C. THC levels are more accurate than THC carboxylic acid levels.
    D. Postmortem plasma levels are more accurate than whole blood.

1769. All of the following are true of dronabinol except _____.

    A. It is a beta-blocker that binds to the CB-1 receptor.
    B. It is approved for chemotherapy-induced nausea.
    C. It is approved for appetite stimulation in AIDS.
    D. It causes a positive result in the urine screening test for marijuana.

1770. The urine metabolite of THC that is usually targeted for screening is _____.

    A. 11-hydroxy-THC
    B. 8-beta-hydroxy-THC

C. 8,11-dehydroxy-THC
D. 11-nor-9-carboxy-THC

1771. All of the following are associated with chronic amphetamine use except _____.

A. permanent neuronal damage
B. glioblastoma
C. vasculitis
D. pulmonary hypertension

1772. The most common illicit drug produced by clandestine labs in the United States is _____.

A. cocaine
B. oxycodone
C. methamphetamine
D. fentanyl

1773. All of the following are indicated in the setting of cocaine-induced acute coronary syndrome except _____.

A. benzodiazepines
B. nitroglycerin
C. beta-adrenergic blockers
D. aspirin

1774. The preferred drug class for the treatment of cocaine-induced narrow complex reentrant supraventricular arrhythmias is _____.

A. calcium channel blockers
B. type IA antiarrhythmics
C. beta-adrenergic blocker
D. type IC antiarrhythmics

1775. If a benzodiazepine fails to sedate an agitated patient using cocaine, the next drug choice would be _____.

   A. haloperidol
   B. promazine
   C. methaqualone
   D. propofol

1776. Ethanol metabolites that are being evaluated as possible makers of previous ethanol use include all of the following except _____.

   A. fatty acid ethyl esters
   B. pyruvate
   C. ethyl sulfate
   D. ethyl glucuronide

1777. All of the following are true regarding the pharmacology of ethanol except _____.

   A. A specific ethanol receptor has recently been identified.
   B. It enhances the inhibitory effects of GABA.
   C. It blocks at the NMDA receptor.
   D. Withdrawal is related to NMDA receptor upregulation.

1778. All of the following are true of the ethanol withdrawal syndrome except _____.

   A. Delirium tremors are the most serious development.
   B. Seizures should be treated with benzodiazepines.
   C. Seizures can be prevented with phenytoin.
   D. Auditory hallucinations can occur.

1779. Disulfiram-type reactions have been reported with all of the following except _____.

   A. cefoperazone
   B. metronidazole

C. chlorpropramide
D. zaleplon

1780. Thiamine deficiency can cause all of the following except
_____.

A. high-output congestive heart failure
B. Wernicke's encephalopathy
C. pulmonary fibrosis
D. Korsakoff's psychosis

1781. In 2007, the adhesive on toy beads that caused an epidemic of
toxicity was chemically related to _____.

A. PCP
B. methamphetamine
C. GHB
D. dextromethorphan

1782. Recreational amyl nitrate inhalant is associated with _____.

A. methemoglobinemia
B. peripheral neuropathy
C. hepatotoxicity
D. renal toxicity

1783. Salvia divinorum is classified as a _____.

A. anticholinergic
B. hallucinogen
C. sympathomimetic
D. THC agonist

1784. GHB is a/an _____.

A. endogenous neurotransmitter
B. releaser of growth hormone

C. a drug of abuse

D. all of the above

1785. The pharmacological effort of Kratom has been related to the presence of _____.

A. safrole

B. atropine

C. salvinorin A

D. mitragynine

1786. The neurobehavioral effects of PCP are most similar to the disease process of _____.

A. mania

B. depression

C. schizophrenia

D. obsessive-compulsive disorder

1787. The mechanism of action of ketamine at clinical concentrations involves _____.

A. binding to the 5HT-2 receptor

B. binding to the 5HT-3 receptor

C. binding to the CB-1 receptor

D. binding to the NMDA receptor

1788. The use of diazepam in the management of chloroquine and cocaine toxicity may involve competitive antagonisms at _____.

A. peripheral benzodiazepine receptors

B. central GABA (A) receptors

C. central GABA (B) receptors

D. central NMDA receptors

1789. All of the following are true of the opiate receptor ORL1 except _____.

A. Nociceptin is an endogenous ligand.
B. It can bind opioid agonists and antagonists.
C. It can be antagonized by naloxone.
D. It has a brain distribution that is similar to other opioid receptor subtypes.

1790. Methylnaltrexone is used to treat opioid-induced _____.

A. respiratory depression
B. nausea
C. sedation
D. constipation

CHAPTER 30 ANSWERS (REFERENCES)

1691. C (I)	1727. C (VI)	1763. A (VI)
1692. A (I)	1728. D (VI)	1764. B (VI)
1693. B (I)	1729. A (VI)	1765. D (VI)
1694. A (I)	1730. C (VI)	1766. C (VIII)
1695. D (I)	1731. A (V)	1767. B (IX)
1696. A (II)	1732. B (VI)	1768. A (IX)
1697. B (III)	1733. A (V)	1769. A (V)
1698. D (I)	1734. D (V)	1770. D (V)
1699. C (I)	1735. C (V)	1771. B (X)
1700. C (I)	1736. A (V)	1772. C (X)
1701. C (III)	1737. C (V)	1773. C (XI)
1702. B (III)	1738. D (V)	1774. A (XI)
1703. B (III)	1739. B (V)	1775. D (XI)
1704. C (III)	1740. C (V)	1776. B (XII)
1705. C (III)	1741. D (VII)	1777. A (XIII)
1706. C (IV)	1742. B (VII)	1778. C (XIV)
1707. D (IV)	1743. C (VII)	1779. D (XV)
1708. B (V)	1744. C (VII)	1780. C (XVI)
1709. A (V)	1745. C (VI)	1781. C (XVII)
1710. D (V)	1746. C (VII)	1782. A (XVIII)
1711. A (VI)	1747. C (VII)	1783. B (XIX)
1712. A (V)	1748. B (VII)	1784. D (XVII)
1713. C (VI)	1749. D (VII)	1785. D (XIX)
1714. B (VI)	1750. B (VII)	1786. C (XX)
1715. D (VI)	1751. A (VI)	1787. D (XX)
1716. B (IV)	1752. C (VI)	1788. A (XXI)
1717. C (IV)	1753. B (VI)	1789. C (XXII)
1718. D (IV)	1754. D (VI)	1790. D (XXIII)
1719. A (IV)	1755. C (VI)	
1720. D (IV)	1756. A (VI)	
1721. A (VI)	1757. D (VI)	
1722. D (VI)	1758. B (VI)	
1723. C (VI)	1759. C (VI)	
1724. D (VI)	1760. A (VI)	
1725. B (VI)	1761. A (VI)	
1726. B (VI)	1762. C (VI)	

REFERENCES

CHAPTER 30

I.   S. B. Karch, "Cocaine," in *Pathology of Drug Abuse*, 4th ed. (Boca Raton: Taylor and Francis, 2009),1–208.

II. Ibid., "Natural Stimulants," in *Pathology of Drug Abuse*, 4th ed. (Boca Raton: Taylor and Francis, 2009), 209–260.

III. Ibid., "Synthetic Stimulants," in *Pathology of Drug Abuse*, 4th ed. (Boca Raton: Taylor and Francis, 2009), 261–312.

IV. Ibid., "Dissociative Anesthetics," in *Pathology of Drug Abuse*, 4th ed. (Boca Raton: Taylor and Francis, 2009), 575–606.

V.   R. B. Swotinsky and D. R. Smith, "Alcohol and Specific Drugs," in *The Medical Review Officer's Manual*, 4th ed.(Beverly Farms: OEM Press, 2010), 217–268.

VI. S. B. Karch, "Opiates and Opioids," in *Pathology of Drug Abuse*, 4th ed. (Boca Raton: Taylor and Francis, 2009), 367–574.

VII. Ibid., "Hallucinogens," in *Pathology of Drug Abuse*, 4th ed. (Boca Raton: Taylor and Francis, 2009), 313–366.

VIII.Ibid., "Anabolic Steroids," in *Pathology of Drug Abuse*, 4th ed. (Boca Raton: Taylor and Francis, 2009), 609–634.

IX. Ibid., "Marijuana," in *Pathology of Drug Abuse*, 4th ed. (Boca Raton: Taylor and Francis, 2009), 649–664.

X.   W. K. Chiang, "Amphetamines," in *Goldfrank's Toxicologic Emergencies*,ed.,ed. L. S. Nelson et al. (New York: McGraw-Hill, 2011), 1078–1090.

XI.   J. M. Prosser and R. S. Hoffman, "Cocaine," in *Goldfrank's Toxicologic Emergencies*, 9th ed., L. S. Nelson et al. (New York: McGraw-Hill, 2011), 1091–1102.

XII.   A. W. Jones, "Biomarkers of Acute and Chronic Alcohol Ingestion," in *Garriott's Medical Legal Aspects of Alcohol*, 5th ed., ed. J. C. Garriott (Tuscon: Lawyers and Judges Publishing Company, 2008), 157–204.

XIII.   L. Yip, "Ethanol," in *Goldfrank's Toxicologic Emergencies*, 9th ed., ed. L. S. Nelson et al. (New York: McGraw-Hill, 2011), 1115–1128.

XIV.   J. A. Gold and L. S. Nelson, "Ethanol Withdrawal," in *Goldfrank's Toxicologic Emergencies*, 9th ed., ed. L. S. Nelson et al. (New York: McGraw-Hill, 2011), 1134–1142.

XV.   L. S. Nelson et al., "Disulfiram and Disulfiram-like Reactions," in *Goldfrank's Toxicologic Emergencies*, 9th ed. (New York: McGraw-Hill, 2011), 1143–1150.

XVI.   R. S. Hoffman, "Thiamine Hydrochloride," in *Goldfrank's Toxicologic Emergencies*, 9th ed., ed. L. S. Nelson et al. (New York: McGraw-Hill, 2011) 1129–1133.

XVII.   B. M. Farmer, "Gamma-Hydroxybutyric Acid," in *Goldfrank's Toxicologic Emergencies*, 9th ed., (New York: McGraw-Hill, 2011), 1151–1156.

XVIII. H. Long, "Inhalants," in *Goldfrank's Toxicologic Emergencies*, 9th ed., ed. L. S. Nelson et al. (New York: McGraw-Hill, 2011), 1157–1165.

XIX.   K. M. Babu, "Hallucinogens," in *Goldfrank's Toxicologic Emergencies*, 9th ed., ed. L. S. Nelson et al. (New York: McGraw-Hill, 2011), 1166–1176.

XX.   R. E. Olmedo, "Phencyclidine and Ketamine," in *Goldfrank's Toxicologic Emergencies*, 9th ed., ed. L. S. Nelson et al. (New York: McGraw-Hill, 2011), 1191–1201.

XXI.   R. S. Hoffman, L. S. Nelson, and M. A. Howland, "Benzodiazepines," in *Goldfrank's Toxicologic Emergencies*, 9th ed., ed. L. S. Nelson et al. (New York: McGraw-Hill, 2011), 1109–114

XXII.   L. S. Nelson and D. Olsen, "Opioids," in *Goldfrank's Toxicologic Emergencies*, 9th ed., ed. L. S. Nelson et al. (New York: McGraw-Hill, 2011), 559–578.

XXIII. M. A. Howland and L. S. Nelson, "Opioid Antagonists," in *Goldfrank's Toxicologic Emergencies*, 9th ed., ed. L. S. Nelson et al. (New York: McGraw-Hill, 2011), 579–585.

31

MEDICAL TOXICOLOGY

1791. If a patient presents to an emergency room with elevated transaminases and an uncertain time of overdose acetaminophen ingestion, the appropriate next step would be _____.

A. Repeat transaminases in 8 hours.
B. Begin N-acetylcysteine.
C. Place patient on transplant list.
D. Obtain liver biopsy.

1792. Which of the following is true regarding acetaminophen overdose during pregnancy?

A. There is no fetal risk because acetaminophen does not cross the placenta.
B. The risk to the fetus from N-acetylcysteine is higher than that from acetaminophen.
C. The risk for fetal liver damage is highest during the first trimester.
D. The fetal liver will have decreased CYP450-medicated metabolism of acetaminophen compared to an adult.

1793. All of the following are true regarding acetaminophen toxicity in alcoholics except _____.

A. The treatment nomogram is modified for alcoholics.
B. The presence of alcohol in the body may be protective.

    C. Chronic alcoholics have induction of CYP2E1.

    D. Alcoholics have decreased glutathione stores because of malnutrition.

1794. All of the following statements are true regarding acetaminophen overdose except _____.

    A. Renal toxicity can occur.

    B. Minor prolongations of the prothrombin time can occur in the absence of hepatotoxicity.

    C. The mortality is less than 0.5 %.

    D. Use of 4 grams acetaminophen per day over 4 weeks is associated with a high risk of hepatoticity.

1795. All of the following are indications for hemodialysis in salicylate overdose except _____.

    A. acute lung injury

    B. hearing loss

    C. renal failure

    D. hepatic injury with coagulopathy

1796. In salicylate toxicity, alkalinization of the serum with intravenous sodium bicarbonate produces all of the following effects except _____.

    A. correction of metabolic acidosis

    B. removal of salicytate from the CNS

    C. enhanced urinary excretion of salicytate

    D. displacement of salicylate from alpha 1 acid glycoprotein

1797. The settings on a ventilator in a salicylite-poisoned patient must be constantly adjusted to maintain preventilator levels of _____.

    A. hypocarbia

    B. oxygen partial pressure

    C. tidal volume

    D. alveolar oxygen

1798. The mechanism for increased cardiovascular risk in users of selective cyclooxygenase 2 inhibitors may involve _____.

A. increased activity of vitamin K–dependant clotting factors
B. decreased fibrinolysis
C. inhibition of endothelial-derived PGI2
D. inhibition of PGE2

1799. The antiplatelet effects of COX-1 inhibitors are due to effects on _____.

A. TXA2
B. PGF
C. PGD
D. leukotrienes

1800. The treatment of intentional nonasprin NSAID overdose usually includes all of the following except _____.

A. serum acetaminophen concentration
B. activated charcoal
C. protein pump inhibitors
D. hemodialysis

1801. The most logical treatment to prevent iron absorption in significant overdose situations is _____.

A. whole-bowel irrigation
B. induced emesis
C. activated charcoal
D. magnesium hydroxide

1802. A rare form of injury from iron overdose that can occur 2 to 8 weeks after ingestion is _____.

A. peripheral neuropathy
B. gastric outlet obstruction
C. pancreatitis
D. bronchiolitis obliterans

1803. The target organ for deferoxamine toxicity is the _____.

    A. liver
    B. lung
    C. kidney
    D. peripheral nervous system

1804. During the 6-hour period following a significant iron overdose, which of the following almost always occurs?

    A. bradycardia
    B. respiratory depression
    C. vomiting
    D. asymptomatic period

1805. All of the following may be indicated in the treatment of vitamin A toxicity except _____.

    A. dexamethasone
    B. intravenous calcium
    C. loop diuretics
    D. activated charcoal

1806. All of the following may be indicated in the treatment of vitamin D overdose except _____.

    A. bisphosphonates
    B. corticosteroids
    C. calcitonin
    D. thiazide diuretics

1807. Neuropathy is mostly likely to be associated with overdose of _____.

    A. vitamin E
    B. vitamin C
    C. pyridoxine
    D. niacin

1808. A coagulopathy is least likely to develop following toxic doses of _____.

A. vitamin A
B. vitamin E
C. pyridoxine
D. niacin

1809. Which of the following best describes the association between vitamin C and risk of oxalate neprolithiasis?

A. It is a significant clinical concern in all patients.
B. It is a significant clinical concern in children and not adults.
C. It is a significant clinical concern in adults and not children.
D. It is not a significant clinical concern.

1810. Which of the following drug classes in an overdose situation is least likely to cause hypoglycemia?

A. first-generation sulfonylureas
B. meglitinides
C. alpha-glucosidase inhibitors
D. second-generation sulfonylureas

1811. Hypoglycemia in the presence of high-insulin plasma levels, high C-peptide plasma levels, and absent insulin-binding antibodies is most likely the result of overdose of _____.

A. exogenous insulin
B. sulfonylureas
C. corticosteroids
D. all of the above

1812. Glucagon is the drug of choice for overdose from _____.

A. sulfonylureas
B. metformin
C. alpha-glucosidase inhibitors
D. none of the above

1813. Overdose of aminoglycosides may produce _____.

   A. aseptic meningitis
   B. acute lung injury
   C. hepatotoxicity
   D. neuromuscular blockade

1814. An unusual adverse effect of fluoroquinolone therapy is _____.

   A. sleep paralysis
   B. nonproductive cough
   C. alopecia
   D. tendon rupture

1815. Lactic acidosis is a serious adverse effect associated with overdose of _____.

   A. nucleoside analog reverse transcriptase inhibitors
   B. penicillin
   C. vancomycin
   D. aminoglycosides

1816. The Jarisch-Herxheimer reaction occurs after administration of _____.

   A. amphotericin B
   B. erythromycin
   C. ciprofloxacin
   D. procaine penicillin G

1817. Which of the following statements is true regarding acute ingestions of long-acting anticoagulant rodenticides?

   A. The risk of coagulation abnormalities is the same in both intentional and small nonintentional overdoses.
   B. Coagulation problems can persist for weeks in intentional overdose.

   C. The 4 hour post-ingestion INR is more clinically relevant than the 48 hour measure.

   D. All children should be hospitalized for 12 hours after a single unintentional dose.

1818. The ideal immediate antidote for life-threatening bleeding in a hemodynamically stable patient with warfarin overdose is _____.

   A. intravenous vitamin K
   B. whole-blood transfusion
   C. prothrombin complex concentrate infusion
   D. fresh frozen plasma infusion

1819. Theoretically, the duration of coagulopathy in long-acting anticoagulant overdose will be shortened by the administration of _____.

   A. phenobarbital
   B. cimetidine
   C. omeprazole
   D. quinine

1820. In patients with gastrointestinal hemorrhage secondary to warfarin-like anticoagulants, the ideal route for vitamin K administrator is _____.

   A. sublingual
   B. intramuscular
   C. subcutaneous
   D. intravenous

1821. All of the following have a place in the treatment of acute thyroid hormone overdose except _____.

   A. high-dose aspirin
   B. acetaminophen
   C. activated charcoal
   D. beta-adrenergic blockers

1822. In patients with asthma, an alternative drug for use in thyroid hormone overdose is _____.

    A. nifidipine
    B. nicardipine
    C. diltiazem
    D. nimodipine

1823. A drug that can sedate a patient with thyroid hormone overdose and also theoretically provide enhanced thyroid elimination is _____.

    A. midazolam
    B. phenobarbital
    C. propofol
    D. mannitol

1824. Which of the following is considered primary therapy for thyroid hormone overdose?

    A. corticosteroids
    B. propylthioiuracil
    C. iodine contrast media
    D. none of the above

1825. All of the following may be indicated in the management of overdose with a histamine 1 receptor antagonist except _____.

    A. lorazepam
    B. physostigmine
    C. warming blankets
    D. sodium bicarbonate

1826. Which of the following is least important in the management of an intentional histamine 1 receptor antagonist overdose?

    A. serum gamma glutamyl transpeptidase
    B. ECG

C. creatine phosphokinase

D. serum acetaminophen level

1827. Oral overdose of histamine 2 receptors antagonists _____.

A. are treated identically as histamine 1 receptor antagonists

B. require orogastric lavage

C. require seizure prophylaxis with phenytoin

D. generally have a good outcome

1828. Which of the following should be avoided in the treatment of decongestant overdose?

A. activated charcoal

B. benzodiazipines

C. phentolamine

D. propranolol

1829. First-line drugs for the treatment of ventricular dysrhythmias from decongestant overdose include _____.

A. verapamil and diltiazem

B. amiodarone and lidocaine

C. quinidine and procainamide

D. atropine and magnesium sulfate

1830. Vasoconstriction from excessive doses of triptan antimigraine therapy can be treated with all of the following except _____.

A. metoprolol

B. phentolamine

C. nitroglycerine

D. sodium nitroprusside

1831. Triptan overdose differs from ergot overdose in that _____.

A. Calcium channel blockers are contraindicated.

B. Vomiting is less.

C. Coronary ischemia does not occur.

D. Diuretics are indicated in the management of hypertension.

1832. Weight loss drugs, methylsergide, and ergotamine have all been associated with _____.

A. amyotropic lateral schlerosis
B. Parkinson's disease
C. myocardial valvular abnormalities
D. hepatic angiosarcoma

1833. Nonanion gap metabolic acidosis is seen following overdose of _____.

A. phenytoin
B. gabapentin
C. topiramate
D. levetiracetam

1834. Which of the following is least likely to cause the drug rash with eosinophilia and systemic symptons (DRESS) syndrome?

A. valproic acid
B. phenytoin
C. carbamazepine
D. primidone

1835. In calcium channel blocker overdose, what serum laboratory parameter may correlate with the severity of poisoning?

A. elevation of potassium
B. decrease in bicarbonate
C. elevation of ionized calcium
D. elevation of glucose

1836. The calcium channel blocker with the most negative ionotropic effect on the heart in overdose is _____.

    A. nicardipine
    B. nifedipine
    C. diltiazem
    D. verapamil

1837. All of the following are true regarding calcium channel blocker overdose except _____.

    A. Nausea and vomiting are common early manifestations.
    B. Hypotension is common.
    C. CNS depression is uncommon without severe hypotension.
    D. All types can produce severe bradycardia in significant overdoses.

1838. All of the following are useful in the treatment of calcium channel blocker overdose except _____.

    A. glucagon
    B. euglycemia insulin therapy
    C. physostigmine
    D. calcium

1839. Patients with a history of sustained release calcium channel blocker ingestion should undergo all of the following except _____.

    A. hospital admission for at least 24 hours
    B. whole bowel irrigation
    C. continuous ECG monitoring
    D. digoxin therapy

1840. In patients overdosing on beta-blockers alone and not taking any comcomittant medication, what property of beta-blockers would render them most toxic?

A. water solubility
B. membrane-stabilizing activity
C. vasodilatory activity
D. cardiac selectivity

1841. Magnesium infusions may be necessary in overdoses of _____.

A. propranolol
B. nadolol
C. sotolol
D. metoprolol

1842. In patients with beta-blocker overdose who do not respond to atropine and fluids, the next drug most recommended for treatment is _____.

A. glucagon
B. theophylline
C. lidocaine
D. dopamine

1843. In beta-blocker overdose with QRS widening, a useful therapy could be _____.

A. hypertonic sodium bicarbonate
B. vasopression
C. potassium
D. isoproterenol

1844. Which of the following has been shown to be the safest beta-blocker in overdose situations?

A. propranolol
B. timolol

C. sotalol

D. atenolol

1845. Naloxone has been used in the treatment of overdoses of _____.

A. clonidine

B. angiotensin-converting enzyme inhibitors

C. ethanol

D. all of the above

1846. In overdoses of direct-acting vasodilators like minoxidil and hydralazine, which peripherally acting alpha-adrenergic agent should be avoided?

A. dopamine

B. norepinephrine

C. phenylephrine

D. all of the above

1847. Newer uses of clonidine that may contribute to a resurgence in cases of toxicity include all of the following except _____.

A. ADHD

B. opioid withdrawal

C. erectile dysfunction

D. nicotine withdrawal

1848. Exposure to nitrous oxide has been associated with all of the following except _____.

A. leukopenia

B. polyneuropathy

C. increased rate of spontaneous abortions

D. scleroderma

1849. Enflurane and desflurane can degrade to _____.

A. CO

B. fluorine gas

C. ozone

D. phosgene

1850. All of the following are true of halothane hepatitis except _____.

A. Eighty percent of cases occur after a single exposure.

B. It is more common in women.

C. There may be a genetic predisposition.

D. Obesity is a risk factor.

1851. Chronic angiotensin receptor blocking therapy can cause hypotension during anesthesia that can be refractory to traditional vasocontrictors, but can respond to _____.

A. ephedrine

B. aldosterone

C. vasopressin

D. glucagon

1852. Hypotension would be least likely following overdose of _____.

A. diazoxide

B. hyrochlorothiazide

C. clonidine

D. nifedipine

1853. All of the following may be helpful in the setting of poisoning with a class 1A antidysrhythmics except _____.

A. flecainide

B. hypertonic sodium bicarbonate

C. magnesium sulfate

D. overdrive pacing

1854. Viscous lidocaine is particularly toxic when swallowed because _____.

A. It has a pleasant taste.

B. It has a high percentage of propylene glycol.

C. It acts as a delayed release form in the gut.

D. The ingestor can receive a very large lidocaine dose.

1855. All of the following may be helpful in the setting of poisoning with a class 1C antidysrhythmics except _____.

A. hypertonic sodium bicarbonate

B. amiodarone

C. cardiopulmonary bypass

D. procainamide

1856. Hyperkalemia during digoxin overdose is best treated with all of the following except _____.

A. dextrose

B. sodium polystyrene sulfonate

C. calcium

D. sodium bicarbonate

1857. The endogenous digoxin-like substance that has been identified in humans is similar to a toxin found in _____.

A. puffer fish

B. potato

C. toads

D. scorpions

1858. Measures to enhance digoxin elimination from the body would include all of the following except _____.

A. activated charcoal

B. acidification of the urine

C. cholestyramine

D. colestipol

1859. Drugs useful in the treatment of dysrhythmias secondary to digoxin overdose include all of the following except _____.

   A. quinidine
   B. lidocaine
   C. phenytoin
   D. atropine

1860. All of the following would be expected to occur following treatment of digoxin toxicity with digoxin-specific Fab except _____.

   A. a decrease in serum-potassium concentration
   B. a decrease in total serum-digoxin concentration
   C. an increase in renal clearance of digoxin
   D. a decrease in free serum-digoxin concentration

1861. In acute digoxin overdose, the best predictor of lethality has been shown to be _____.

   A. serum-potassium concentration
   B. serum-total digoxin concentration
   C. PR interval
   D. serum-free digoxin concentration

1862. All of the following are useful in the treatment of hemodynamically unstable ventricular tachycardia secondary to digoxin overdose except _____.

   A. lidocaine
   B. digoxin-specific Fab
   C. cardioversion
   D. transvenous pacemaker overdrive suppression

1863. A distinguishing feature of the serotonin syndrome from the neuroleptic malignant syndrome is _____.

   A. altered mental status
   B. elevated core temperature

C. tachycardia

D. myoclonus

1864. All of the following could be useful in the treatment of severe neuroleptic malignant syndrome except _____.

A. acidification of urine

B. dantrolene

C. prophylactic-dose, low-molecular-weight heparin

D. benzodiazepines

1865. All of the following are appropriate in the management of acute antipsychotic overdose except _____.

A. intravenous fluids

B. syrup of ipecac

C. activated charcoal

D. cardiac monitoring

1866. The antipsychotic with the highest degree of QT prolongation is _____.

A. aripiprazole

B. olanzapine

C. thioridazine

D. risperidone

1867. The antipsychotic with the lowest incidence of tardive dyskinesia is _____.

A. haloperidol

B. fluphenazine

C. chlorpromazine

D. clozapine

1868. All of the following are useful in eliminating drug from carbamazipine overdose except _____.

A. multiple-dose activated charcoal
B. urine alkalinization
C. hemodialysis
D. charcoal hemoperfusion

1869. Cardiac toxicity from intravenous phenytoin preparations is thought to be due in part to _____.

A. phenytoin-degradation products
B. oxalic acid
C. propylene glycol
D. cetyl alcohol

1870. A predictor of persistent neurologic dysfunction in patients with lithium toxicity is _____.

A. elevated creatinine
B. polyuria
C. hyperpyrexia
D. hypothyroidisim

1871. The recommended treatment for gastrointestinal lithium elimination after ingestion of sustained release preparations is _____.

A. whole-bowel irrigation
B. multiple-dose activated charcoal
C. orogastric lavage
D. cholestyramine

1872. Hemodialysis should be considered in the management of patients with lithium toxicity and concurrent _____.

A. severe neurotoxicity
B. renal failure and neurotoxicity

C. congestive heart failure

D. all of the above

1873. A treatment that has no role in the management of a patient with lithium toxicity is _____.

A. peritoneal dialysis

B. saline infusion

C. continuous renal replacement therapy (CRRT)

D. all of the above

1874. Toxicity may develop because of a drug interaction between lithium and _____.

A. thiazide diuretics

B. angiotensin converting enzyme inhibitors

C. NSAIDs

D. all of the above

1875. All of the following are indicated in monoamine oxidase inhibitor–induced serotonin syndrome except _____.

A. dopamine

B. cooling measures

C. benzodiazipines

D. cyproheptadine

1876. Serious drug interactions can occur between monoamine oxidase inhibitors and all of the following except _____.

A. dextromethorphan

B. tramadol

C. acetaminophen

D. meperidine

1877. The interaction of tyramine in food with first-generation monoamine oxidase inhibitors produces _____.

    A. serotonin syndrome
    B. malignant neuroleptic syndrome
    C. hyperadrenergic crisis
    D. all of the above

1878. The hyperthermia from monoamine oxidase–induced serotonin syndrome is best treated with _____.

    A. acetaminophen
    B. phenothiazines
    C. dantrolene
    D. none of the above

1879. Seizures refractory to benzodiazepines following large overdoses of phenelzine should be treated with _____.

    A. pyridoxine
    B. phenytoin
    C. aripiprazole
    D. none of the above

1880. A unique toxicity of trazodone is _____.

    A. inhibition of CYP2C19
    B. hypothyroidism
    C. cholestatic hepatitis
    D. priapism

1881. The drug most commonly associated with the drug discontinuation syndrome is _____.

    A. paroxetine
    B. venlafaxine
    C. fluoxetine
    D. trazodone

1882. The SSRI with the highest incidence of QT prolongation is
_____.

    A. sertraline
    B. paroxetine
    C. citalopram
    D. fluoxetine

1883. The SSRI with the highest incidence of seizures is _____.

    A. sertraline
    B. escitalopram
    C. fluvoxamine
    D. fluoxetine

1884. An atypical antidepressant with a low incidence of seizures is
_____.

    A. bupropion
    B. trazodone
    C. duloxetine
    D. venlafaxine

1885. Patients die from cyclic antidepressant overdose primarily as a
result of _____.

    A. central nervous system toxicity
    B. cardiovascular toxicity
    C. anticholinergic toxicity
    D. pulmonary toxicity

1886. Risk factors for the development of ventricular tachycardia
during tricyclic antidepressant overdose include all of the
following except _____.

    A. hypoxia
    B. acidosis
    C. beta-adrenergic agonist concurrent therapy
    D. beta-adrenergic antagonist concurrent therapy

1887. Life-threatening toxicity from tricyclic antidepressant overdose usually occurs with levels at or above _____.

    A. 10 ng/mL
    B. 100 ng/mL
    C. 200 ng/mL
    D. 1,000 ng/mL

1888. All of the following have a role in the management of cyclic antidepressant toxicity except _____.

    A. dantrolene
    B. sodium bicarbonate
    C. benzodiazepines
    D. magnesium sulfate

1889. The cyclic antidepressant with a lower incidence of serious cardiac toxicity, but a higher incidence of seizures is _____.

    A. nortriptyline
    B. protriptyline
    C. amoxapine
    D. imipramine

1890. Significant dermal absorption can occur after exposure to _____.

    A. chlorhexidine
    B. benzalkonium chloride
    C. sodium hypochlorite
    D. phenol

1891. The "boiled lobster rash" is characteristic of ingestion of _____.

    A. glutaraldehyde
    B. boric acid
    C. sodium chlorate
    D. formaldehyde

1892. Lavage with a starch solution may be useful in preventing toxicity from oral ingestion of products containing _____.

A. iodine
B. potassium permanganate
C. sodium hypochlorite
D. boric acid

1893. Oxygen embolus is a toxic effect from poisoning with _____.

A. potassium permanganate
B. glutaraldehyde
C. hydrogen peroxide
D. sodium hypochlorite

1894. Methemoglobinemia may result from ingestion of _____.

A. phenol and sodium chlorate
B. mercurochrome and thimerosal
C. hexachlorophene and benzalkonium chloride
D. isopropanol and boric acid

1895. Orogastric lavage is possibly indicated for all of the following hydrocarbon ingestions except _____.

A. camphor
B. carbon tetrachloride
C. those associated with spontaneous vomiting
D. benzene

1896. Which of the following is indicated in the initial management of nearly all hydrocarbon ingestions?

A. corticosteroids
B. prophylactic antibiotics
C. benzodiazepines
D. none of the above

1897. All of the following would be indicated in a patient with hematemesis secondary to methylxanthine toxicity except _____.

A. cimetidine
B. ranitidine
C. pantoprazole
D. omeprazole

1898. Seizures from methylxanthine toxicity can be treated with all of the following except _____.

A. benzodiazepines
B. barbiturates
C. phenytoin
D. propofol

1899. Which of the following drugs would be inappropriate for the treatment of supraventricular arrhythymias from methylxanthine overdose?

A. benzodiazipines
B. esmolol
C. verapamil
D. physostigmine

1900. Toxicity from methylxanthine involves all of the following activities except _____.

A. inhibition of phosphodiesterase
B. stimulation at beta-adrenergic receptors
C. antagonism at adenosine receptors
D. nicotinic cholinergic receptor blockade

1901. All of the following are effective ways to enhance the elimination of methylxanthines except _____.

A. urinary acidification
B. hemodialysis

C. charcoal hemoperfusion

D. multiple-dose activated charcoal

1902. The most common form of toxicity from beta-2 selective adrenergic agonist overdose is from children ingesting oral _____.

A. terbutaline

B. albuterol

C. clenbuterol

D. salmeterol

1903. All of the following are suggested indications for hyperbaric oxygen therapy in carbon monoxide poisoning except _____.

A. duration of exposure of 24 hours or longer

B. unconsciousness

C. age less than 36 years

D. COHb level greater than 30 %

1904. The most significant toxicity with carbon monoxide poisoning is _____.

A. delayed neurologic or neuropsychiatric sequelae

B. seizures

C. acute lung injury

D. cardiomyopathy

1905. Which of the following chemical–chemical weapon class pairs is incorrect?

A. 1-chloracetophenone–riot control agent

B. phosgene–nerve gas

C. lewisite-vesicant

D. 3 quinuclidinyl benzilate–incapacitating agent

1906. The most serious common consequence of camphor ingestion is _____.

    A. seizure
    B. toxic shock syndrome
    C. hepatic necrosis
    D. esophageal perforation

1907. All of the following are true of succimer except _____.

    A. It can be given orally.
    B. It can be co-administered with iron.
    C. It is used for lead, mercury, and arsenic toxicity.
    D. It is contraindicated in G6PD-deficient patients.

1908. An association between denture creams and neurologic toxicity has recently been described which is presumed to be due to an excess of _____.

    A. zinc
    B. copper
    C. chromium
    D. selenium

1909. All of the following can cause an increased osmol gap except_____.

    A. methanol
    B. asprin
    C. ethanol
    D. isopropanol

1910. All of the following can cause a primary metabolic acidosis except ____.

    A. quinidine
    B. paraldehyde
    C. toluene
    D. iron

1911. Methylsalicylate has a characteristic odor of_____.

    A. vinyl
    B. garlic
    C. wintergreen
    D. bitter almonds

1912. A patient who overdoses on a drug with a significant enterohepatic recirculation and the formation of active recirculating metabolites would most benefit from _____.

    A. dialysis
    B. multiple-dose activated charcoal
    C. exchange transfusion
    D. phenobarbital

1913. Which of the following procedures to enhance poison elimination has fallen out of favor?

    A. alkalinization of urine
    B. dialysis
    C. multiple-dose activated charcoal
    D. acidification of urine

1914. The major concern with intravenous administration of N-acetylcysteine is _____.

    A. anaphylactoid reaction
    B. vein phlebitis
    C. hypotension
    D. cardiac arrhythmia

1915. A cofactor used in the treatment of methanol overdose is _____.

    A. thiamine
    B. vitamin B_{12}
    C. folic acid
    D. pyridoxine

1916. The ECG parameter that correlates best with severity in a tricyclic antidepressant overdose is _____.

   A. PR interval
   B. heart rate
   C. ORS interval
   D. T wave height

1917. Patients with significant caustic ingestion are at an increased risk of all of the following except _____.

   A. esophageal stricture
   B. esophageal carcinoma
   C. esophageal varices
   D. esophageal perforation

CHAPTER 31 ANSWERS (REFERENCES)

1791. B (I)	1827. D (X)	1863. D (XIX)
1792. D (I)	1828. D (X)	1864. A (XIX)
1793. A (I)	1829. B (X)	1865. B (XIX)
1794. D (I)	1830. A (XI)	1866. C (XIX)
1795. B (II)	1831. B (XI)	1867. D (XIX)
1796. D (II)	1832. C (XI)	1868. B (XII)
1797. A (II)	1833. C (XII)	1869. C (XII)
1798. C (III)	1834. A (XII)	1870. C (XX)
1799. A (III)	1835. D (XIII)	1871. A (XX)
1800. D (III)	1836. D (XIII)	1872. D (XX)
1801. A (IV)	1837. A (XIII)	1873. A (XX)
1802. B (IV)	1838. C (XIII)	1874. D (XX)
1803. B (IV)	1839. D (XIII)	1875. A (XXI)
1804. C (IV)	1840. B (XIV)	1876. C (XXI)
1805. B (V)	1841. C (XIV)	1877. C (XXI)
1806. D (V)	1842. A (XIV)	1878. D (XXI)
1807. C (V)	1843. A (XIV)	1879. A (XXI)
1808. C (V)	1844. D (XIV)	1880. D (XXII)
1809. D (V)	1845. D (XV)	1881. A (XXII)
1810. C (VI)	1846. A (XVI)	1882. C (XXII)
1811. B (VI)	1847. C (XVI)	1883. B (XXII)
1812. D (VI)	1848. D (XXXIV)	1884. B (XXII)
1813. D (VII)	1849. A (XXXIV)	1885. B (XXII)
1814. D (VII)	1850. A (XXXIV)	1886. D (XXIII)
1815. A (VII)	1851. C (XVI)	1887. D (XXIII)
1816. D (VII)	1852. B (XVI)	1888. A (XXIII)
1817. B (VIII)	1853. A (XVII)	1889. C (XXIII)
1818. C (VIII)	1854. D (XVII)	1890. D (XXIV)
1819. A (VIII)	1855. D (XVII)	1891. B (XXIV)
1820. C (VIII)	1856. C (XVIII)	1892. A (XXIV)
1821. A (IX)	1857. C (XVIII)	1893. C (XXIV)
1822. C (IX)	1858. B (XVIII)	1894. A (XXIV)
1823. B (IX)	1859. A (XVIII)	1895. C (XXV)
1824. D (IX)	1860. B (XVIII)	1896. D (XXV)
1825. C (X)	1861. A (XVIII)	1897. A (XXVI)
1826. A (X)	1862. D (XVIII)	1898. C (XXVI)

1899. D (XXVI)
1900. D (XXVI)
1901. A (XXVI)
1902. B (XXVI)
1903. C (XXVII)
1904. A (XXVII)
1905. B (XXVIII)
1906. A (XXIX)
1907. D (XXX)
1908. A (XXXI)
1909. B (XXXII)
1910. A (XXXII)
1911. C (XXXII)
1912. B (XXXII)
1913. D (XXXII)
1914. A (XXXII)
1915. C (XXXII)
1916. C (XXXII)
1917. C (XXXIII)

REFERENCES

CHAPTER 31

I. R. G. Hendrickson, "Acetaminophen," in *Goldfrank's Toxicologic Emergencies*, 9th ed., ed. L. S. Nelson et al. (New York: McGraw-Hill, 2011), 483–499.

II. N. E. Flomenbaum, "Salicylates," in *Goldfrank's Toxicologic Emergencies*, 9th ed., ed. L. S. Nelson et al. (New York: McGraw-Hill, 2011), 508–521.

III. W. J. Holubek, "Nonsteroidal Anti-inflammatory Drugs," in *Goldfrank's Toxicologic Emergencies*, 9th ed., ed. L. S. Nelson et al. (New York: McGraw-Hill, 2011), 528–536.

IV. J. Perrone, "Iron," in *Goldfrank's Toxicologic Emergencies*, 9th ed., ed. L. S. Nelson et al. (New York: McGraw-Hill, 2011), 596–603.

V. G. Y. Ginsberg, "Vitamins," in *Goldfrank's Toxicologic Emergencies*, 9th ed., ed. L. S. Nelson et al. (New York: McGraw-Hill, 2011), 609–623.

VI. G. M. Bosse, "Antidiabetic and Hypoglycemics," in *Goldfrank's Toxicologic Emergencies*, 9th ed., ed. L. S. Nelson et al. (New York: McGraw-Hill, 2011), 714–727.

VII. C. M. Stork, "Antibacterials, Antifungals, and Antimalerials," in *Goldfrank's Toxicologic Emergencies*, 9th ed., ed. L. S. Nelson et al. (New York: McGraw-Hill, 2011),817–833.

VIII. M. Su, "Anticoagulants," in *Goldfrank's Toxicologic Emergencies*, 9th ed., ed. L. S. Nelson et al. (New York: McGraw-Hill, 2011), 861-875.

IX. N. C. Bouchard, "Thyroid and Antithyroid Medication," in *Goldfrank's Toxicologic Emergencies*, 9th ed., ed. L. S. Nelson et al. (New York: McGraw-Hill, 2011), 738–747.

X. A. J. Yomassoni and R. S. Weisman, "Antihistamines and Decongestants," in *Goldfrank's Toxicologic Emergencies*, 9th ed., ed. L. S. Nelson et al. (New York: McGraw-Hill, 2011), 748–758.

XI. J. Chu, "Antimigraine Medications," in *Goldfrank's Toxicologic Emergencies*, 9th ed., ed. L. S. Nelson et al. (New York: McGraw-Hill, 2011), 763–769.

XII. S. Doyon, "Anticonvulsants," in *Goldfrank's Toxicologic Emergencies*, 9th ed., ed. L. S. Nelson et al. (New York: McGraw-Hill, 2011), 698–710.

XIII. F. J. DeRoos, "Calcium Channel Blockers," in *Goldfrank's Toxicologic Emergencies*, 9th ed., ed. L. S. Nelson et al. (New York: McGraw-Hill, 2011), 884–892.

XIV. J. R. Brubacher, "β-Adrenergic Antagonists," in *Goldfrank's Toxicologic Emergencies*, 9th ed., ed. L. S. Nelson et al. (New York: McGraw-Hill, 2011), 896–909.

XV. M. A. Howland and L. S. Nelson, "Opioid Antagonists," in *Goldfrank's Toxicologic Emergencies*, 9th ed., ed. L. S. Nelson et al. (New York: McGraw-Hill, 2011), 579–585.

XVI. F. J. DeRoos, "Other Antihypertensives," in *Goldfrank's Toxicologic Emergencies*, 9th ed., ed. L. S. Nelson et al. (New York: McGraw-Hill, 2011), 914–924.

XVII. L. S. Nelson and N. A. Lewin, "Antidysrhythmics," in *Goldfrank's Toxicologic Emergencies*, 9th ed., ed. L. S. Nelson et al. (New York: McGraw-Hill, 2011), 925–935.

XVIII. J. Hack, "Cardioactive Steroids," in *Goldfrank's Toxicologic Emergencies*, 9th ed., ed. L. S. Nelson et al. (New York: McGraw-Hill, 2011), 936–945.

XIX. D. N. Juurlink, "Antipsychotics," in *Goldfrank's Toxicologic Emergencies*, 9th ed., ed. L. S. Nelson et al. (New York: McGraw-Hill, 2011), 1003–1015.

XX.   H. A. Greller, "Lithium," in *Goldfrank's Toxicologic Emergencies*, 9th ed., ed. L. S. Nelson et al. (New York: McGraw-Hill, 2011),1016–1026.

XXI.   A. F. Manini, "Monoamine Oxidase Inhibitors," in *Goldfrank's Toxicologic Emergencies*, 9th ed., ed. L. S. nelson et al. (New York: McGraw-Hill, 2011),1027–1036.

XXII.   C. M. Stork, "Serotonin Reuptake Inhibitors and Atypical Antidepressants," in *Goldfrank's Toxicologic Emergencies*, 9th ed., ed. L. S. Nelson et al. (New York: McGraw-Hill, 2011),1037–1048.

XXIII. E. L. Liebelt, "Cyclic Antidepressants," in *Goldfrank's Toxicologic Emergencies*, 9th ed., ed. L. S. Nelson et al. (New York: McGraw-Hill, 2011),1049–1059.

XXIV.   P. M. Wax, "Antiseptics, Disinfectants, and Sterilants," in *Goldfrank's Toxicologic Emergencies*, 9th ed., ed. L. S. Nelson et al. (New York: McGraw-Hill, 2011),1345–1357.

XXV.   D. D. Gummin, "Hydrocarbons," in *Goldfrank's Toxicologic Emergencies*, 9th ed., ed. L. S. Nelson et al. (New York: McGraw-Hill, 2011), 1386–1399.

XXVI.   R.J.Hoffman,"MethylxanthinesandSelectiveBeta-2Adrenergic Agonists," in *Goldfrank's Toxicologic Emergencies*, 9th ed., ed. L. S. Nelson et al. (New York: McGraw-Hill, 2011), 952–964.

XXVII. C. Tomaszewski, "Carbon Monoxide," in *Goldfrank's Toxicologic Emergencies*, 9th ed., ed. L. S. Nelson et al. (New York: McGraw-Hill, 2011),1658–1670.

XXVIII. J. R. Suchard, "Chemical Weapons," in *Goldfrank's Toxicologic Emergencies*, 9th ed., ed. L. S. Nelson et al. (New York: McGraw-Hill, 2011),1735–1749.

XXIX. E. K. Kuffner, "Camphor and Moth Repellents," in *Goldfrank's Toxicologic Emergencies*, 9th ed., ed. L. S. Nelson et al. (New York: McGraw-Hill, 2011),1358–1363.

XXX. M. A. Howland, "Succimer (2,3-dimercaptosuccinic acid)," in *Goldfrank's Toxicologic Emergencies*, 9th ed., ed. L. S. Nelson et al. (New York: McGraw-Hill, 2011),1284–1289.

XXXI. N. Majlesi, "Zinc," in *Goldfrank's Toxicologic Emergencies*, 9th ed., ed. L. S. Nelson et al. (New York: McGraw-Hill, 2011), 1339–1344.

XXXII. L. R. Cantilena, "Clinical Toxicology," in *Casarett & Doull's Toxicology: The Basic Science of Poisons*, 7th ed., ed. L. S. Nelson et al. (New York: McGraw-Hill, 2008),1257–1272.

XXXIII. J. A. Fulton, "Caustics," in *Goldfrank's Toxicologic Emergencies*, 9th ed., ed. L. S. Nelson et al. (New York: McGraw-Hill, 2011), 1364–1373.

XXXIV. B. Kaufman and M. Griffel, "Inhalational Anesthetics," in *Goldfrank's Toxicologic Emergencies*, 9th ed., ed. L. S. Nelson et al. (New York: McGraw-Hill, 2011), 982-988.

32

EPIDEMIOLOGY/ STATISTICS/RISK ASSESSMENT

1918. Incidence rate is _____.

A. number of subjects with an abnormality at a specified time
B. number of subjects developing an abnormality per population within a specific time interval
C. number of subjects with an abnormality divided by the number of subjects without the abnormality
D. number of subjects with an abnormality divided by the total number of subjects

1919. The statistical test used to determine whether there is an association between cigarette smoking and bladder cancer by comparing the number of cases of cancer in smokers vs. nonsmokers to smokers vs. nonsmokers without cancer in the same population would be _____.

A. 1-tablet t-test
B. 2-tablet t-test
C. analysis of variance
D. chi-square test

1920. The statistical test used to determine whether 3 different doses of a new antihypertensive medicine work better than placebo would be _____.

A. 2 sample t-test
B. paired t-test
C. analysis of variance
D. chi-square test

1921. The statistical test used to determine whether rheumatoid arthritis has an effect on the urinary excretion of X would be _____.

A. 2 sample t-test
B. paired t-test
C. analysis of variance
D. chi-square test

1922. Three standard deviations on either side of the mean account for what percent of the population?

A. 90 %
B. 95 %
C. 97 %
D. greater than 99 %

1923. The quantity that assesses uncertainty in a population mean is _____.

A. SD
B. SEM
C. F statistic
D. p-value

1924. Statistical tests for continuous data include all of the following except _____.

A. chi-square
B. paired t-test

    C. 2 sample t-test

    D. analysis of variance

1925. Data that is measured on an arithmetic scale is considered _____.

    A. nominal

    B. ordinal

    C. continuous

    D. integer

1926. The square root of a sample's variance is _____.

    A. SD

    B. SEM

    C. F statistic

    D. P value

1927. The F statistic is used in _____.

    A. chi-square test

    B. ANOVA

    C. 2 sample t-test

    D. paired t-test

1928. The probability of observing a particular study result by chance alone when the null hypothesis is really true is _____.

    A. T value

    B. N value

    C. relative risk

    D. P valve

1929. A study in which a disease-free group exposed to X is followed prospectively to determine whether a disease occurs at a different rate compared to a nonexposed group in _____.

    A. case-controlled study

    B. phase 1 clinical trial

    C. cohort study
    D. phase 4 clinical trial

1930. A retrospective study that compares a group of subjects with a disease to a group of subjects without the disease is _____.

    A. case-controlled study
    B. phase 2 clinical trial
    C. cohort study
    D. phase 3 clinical trial

1931. The relative risk is calculated from the results of _____.

    A. case-controlled study
    B. cohort study
    C. matched case-control study
    D. all of the above

1932. The odds ratio is an estimation of the_____.

    A. p-value
    B. confidence interval
    C. relative risk
    D. F statistic

1933. The rate of an event in an exposed population minus the rate in a nonexposed population is called _____.

    A. absolute risk
    B. relative risk
    C. attributable risk
    D. real risk

1934. The disease rate in an exposed group divided by the disease rate in a nonexposed group is called _____.

    A. odds ratio
    B. relative risk

    C. absolute risk

    D. prevalence

1935. The null hypothesis means _____.

    A. There is no difference between the groups.

    B. There is a certain probability of a difference between the groups.

    C. There is a difference between the groups.

    D. none of the above

1936. A type 1 error _____.

    A. rejects the null hypothesis when the groups are really different

    B. misses a real difference between 2 groups

    C. does not reject the null hypothesis when the groups are really different

    D. rejects the null hypothesis when the groups are really the same

1937. A systematic difference other than treatment between 2 groups is called ____.

    A. chance

    B. confidence level

    C. randomness

    D. bias

1938. The probability that there is not a type II error is called _____.

    A. power

    B. degree of freedom

    C. sensitivity

    D. robustness

1939. Body weights of a 21-year-old male will follow a _____ distribution.

A. normal
B. bimodal
C. skewed
D. ranked

1940. A parameter that shows the degree of statistical relationship between the variables in 2 groups is called _____.

A. power
B. robustness
C. correlation coefficient
D. specificity

1941. An analysis of several separate but similar studies to produce a single result is called _____.

A. linear regression analysis
B. least squares analysis
C. Monte Carlo analysis
D. Meta-analysis

1942. True positives divided the sum of true positives and false negatives is _____.

A. positive predictive value
B. sensitivity
C. negative predictive value
D. specificity

1943. True negatives divided by the sum of false positives and true negatives is _____.

A. positive predictive value
B. sensitivity
C. negative predictive value
D. specificity

1944. True positives divided by the sum of true positives and false positives is _____.

A. positive predictive value
B. sensitivity
C. negative predictive value
D. specificity

1945. True negatives divided by the sum of false negatives and true negatives is _____.

A. positive predictive value
B. sensitivity
C. negative predictive value
D. specificity

1946. A factor that is associated with the exposure of interest and is also an independent cause of the disease being studied is called a/an _____.

A. independent variable
B. dependent variable
C. false assumption
D. confounder

1947. The ratio of observed to expected deaths in a study is called _____.

A. proportional mortality ratio
B. standardized mortality ratio
C. morbidity ratio
D. life expectancy ratio

1948. On a dose-response curve, the highest nonstatistically significant dose tested is called _____.

A. LOAEL
B. NOAEL

C. reference dose

D. point of departure

1949. On a dose-response curve, the lowest dose tested with a statistically significant effect is _____.

A. LOAEL

B. NOAEL

C. reference dose

D. point of departure

1950. The epidemiological study design most suitable for the study of rare diseases is _____.

A. clinical trial

B. cohort

C. case control

D. cross-sectional

1951. Assessing the chemical structure of a toxic molecule to predict toxicity in other similar molecules is called _____.

A. molecular orbital correlations

B. steriochemical predictiveness

C. quantum toxicology

D. structure-activity relationships

1952. A threshold for toxicity is assumed for all of the following toxicants except _____.

A. teratogens

B. carcinogens

C. hepatotoxins

D. skeletal muscle toxins

CHAPTER 32 ANSWERS (REFERENCES)

1918. B (I)
1919. D (I)
1920. C (I)
1921. A (I)
1922. D (I)
1923. B (I)
1924. A (I)
1925. C (I)
1926. A (I)
1927. B (I)
1928. D (I)
1929. C (I)
1930. A (I)
1931. B (I)
1932. C (I)
1933. C (I)
1934. B (I)
1935. A (I)
1936. D (I)
1937. D (II)
1938. A (II)
1939. A (II)
1940. C (II)
1941. D (II)
1942. B (III)
1943. D (III)
1944. A (III)
1945. C (III)
1946. D (I)
1947. B (I)
1948. B (IV)
1949. A (IV)
1950. C (IV)
1951. D (IV)
1952. B (IV)

REFERENCES

CHAPTER 32

I.   M. B. Schenker, "Biostatistics and Epidemiology," in *Current Occupational and Environmental Medicine*, 4th ed., ed. J. Landou (New York: McGraw-Hill, 2007), 789–812.

II.   S. C. Gad, "Statistics for Toxicologists," in *Principles and Methods of Toxicology*, 5th ed., ed. A. W. Hayes (Boca Raton: Taylor and Francis, 2008), 369–452.

III.   R. R. Cook, "Epidemiology for Toxicologists," in *Principles and Methods of Toxicology*, 5th ed., ed. A. W. Hayes (Boca Raton: Taylor and Francis, 2008), 549–590.

IV.   E. M. Faustman and G. S. Omenn, "Risk Assessment," in *Casarett & Doull's Toxicology: The Basic Science of Poisons*, 7th ed., ed. C. D. Klaassen (New York: McGraw-Hill, 2008), 107–128.

33

ALCOHOL TOXICOLOGY

1953. To convert a serum alcohol concentration to an approximate blood alcohol concentration (BAC), one should _____.

A. Divide the serum level by the hematocrit.
B. Multiply the serum level by 1.45.
C. Divide the serum level by 1.15.
D. Multiply the serum level by the hematocrit.

1954. Which of the following substances will affect the one leg standing (OLS) field sobriety test _____.

A. stimulants
B. inhalants
C. hallucinogens
D. all of the above

1955. The blood alcohol concentration (BAC) to breath alcohol concentration ratio is normally considered to be approximately _____.

A. 250
B. 2,100
C. 1
D. 4,500

1956. All of the following are considered field sobriety tests except
_____.

A. whisper hearing
B. one leg standing
C. horozonal gaze nystagmus
D. walk and turn

1957. Which of the following could cause a false positive blood
alcohol level as high as 40 mg/dL?

A. use of isopropyl alcohol swab
B. sorbitol use
C. recent ingestion of green tea
D. none of the above

1958. The range of alcohol elimination from a normal healthy adult
is considered to be _____.

A. 1 to 2 mg/dL/hr
B. 1 to 2 gm/L/hr
C. 14 to 17 gm/L/hr
D. 14 to 17 mg/dL/hr

1959. The volume of distribution of ethyl alcohol in a healthy
nonobese adult is normally considered to be _____.

A. 0.2 to 0.3 L/kg
B. 0.3 to 0.5 L/kg
C. 0.60 to 0.70 L/kg
D. 1.2 to 1.5 L/kg

1960. A postmortem blood alcohol level done on femerol blood taken
4 hours after death is considered to be _____.

A. approximately equal to the level at the time of death
B. falsely low by at least 50 %

C. falsely high by at least 50 %

D. subject to drug interactions that would not occur during life

1961. A 170-pound healthy male with a blood alcohol level of 55 mg/dL would have most likely consumed ____ standard drinks over 1 hour.

A. 1
B. 2.5
C. 4.5
D. 6

1962. At a blood alcohol concentration of 140 mg/dL, the relative probability of being involved in a car accident is increased ____ fold.

A. 5
B. 10
C. 15
D. 20

1963. The number of grams of ethanol in a standard drink in the United States is approximately ____.

A. 5
B. 7
C. 14
D. 20

1964. The density of ethanol is ____.

A. 0.58 g/mL
B. 0.79 g/mL
C. 0.94 g/mL
D. 1.08 g/mL

1965. The Widmark equation is used to calculate _____.

    A. amount of equilibrated alcohol at time of blood sampling
    B. ethanol's elimination rate constant
    C. ethanol's absorption rate constant
    D. ethanol's distribution rate constant

1966. The liver enzyme that is the most sensitive as a biomarker for ethanol abuse is _____.

    A. gamma glutamyl transferase (GGT)
    B. alkaline phosphatase
    C. aspartate aminotransferase (AST)
    D. alanine aminotransferase (ALT)

1967. In a decomposed or embalmed body, the specimen to use to measure an alcohol level that would best correlate with a blood alcohol is _____.

    A. hair
    B. bone marrow
    C. skin
    D. vitreous humor

CHAPTER 33 ANSWERS (REFERENCES)

1953. C (I)
1954. D (II)
1955. B (III)
1956. A (II)
1957. D (I)
1958. D (IV)
1959. C (IV)
1960. A (V)
1961. B (IV)
1962. D (II)
1963. C (VI)
1964. B (IV)
1965. A (IV)
1966. A (VII)
1967. D (V)

REFERENCES

CHAPTER 33

I. Y. H. Caplan and B. A. Goldberger, "Blood, Urine, and Other Fluid and Tissue Specimens for Alcohol Analysis," in *Garriott's Medicolegal Aspects of Alcohol*, 5th ed., ed. J. C. Garriott (Tuscon: Lawyers and Judges Publishing Company, 2008), 205–216.

II. J. E. Manno, B. R. Manno, and K. E. Ferslaw, "Experimental Basis of Alcohol Psychomotor Performance," in *Garriott's Medicolegal Aspects of Alcohol*, 5th ed., ed. J. C. Garriott (Tuscon: Lawyers and Judges Publishing Company, 2008), 347–378.

III. P. Harding and R. Zettl, "Methods for Breath Analysis," in *Garriott's Medicolegal Aspects of Alcohol*, 5th ed., ed. J. C. Garriott (Tuscon: Lawyers and Judges Publishing Company, 2008), 229–254.

IV. A. W. Jones, "Biochemical and Physiological Research on the Disposition and Fate of Ethanol in the Body," in *Garriott's Medicolegal Aspects of Alcohol*, 5th ed., ed. J. C. Garriott (Tuscon: Lawyers and Judges Publishing Company, 2008), 47–156.

V. J. C. Garriott, "Analysis for Alcohol in Post Mortem Specimens," in *Garriott's Medicolegal Aspects of Alcohol*, 5th ed. (Tuscon: Lawyers and Judges Publishing Company, 2008), 217–228.

VI. B. H. McAnalley and E. H. Aguayo, "Chemistry of Alcoholic Beverages," in *Garriott's Medicolegal Aspects of Alcohol*, 5th ed., ed. J. C. Garriott (Tuscon: Lawyers and Judges Publishing Company, 2008), 1–25.

VII. A. W. Jones, "Biomarkers of Acute and Chronic Alcohol Ingestion," in *Garriott's Medicolegal Aspects of Alcohol*, 5th ed., ed. J. C. Garriott (Tuscon: Lawyers and Judges Publishing Company, 2008), 157–204.

34

ANTIDOTES

Matching Test

1968. sodium bicarbonate

1969. L-carnitine

1970. intravenous fat emulsion

1971. glucagon

1972. octreotide

1973. dantrolene sodium

1974. Prussian blue

1975. physostigmine

1976. protamine

1977. pyridoxine

1978. leucovorin

1979. flumazenil

1980. fomepizole

1981. benzodiazepines

1982. atropine

1983. calcium

1984. pentate zinc trisodium

A. methotrexate

B. cholinesterase inhibitor

C. isoniazid

D. heparin

E. thallium

F. bupivacaine

G. ethanol withdrawal

H. valproic acid toxicity

I. plutonium

J. hydrogen fluoride

K. anticholinergic toxicity

L. beta-adrenergic antagonists

M. ethylene glycol

N. malignant hyperthermia

O. midazolam

P. sulfonylurea-induced hypoglycemia

Q. cyclic antidepressants

CHAPTER 34 ANSWERS (REFERENCES)

1968. Q (I)

1969. H (II)

1970. F (III)

1971. L (IV)

1972. P (V)

1973. N (VI)

1974. E (VII)

1975. K (VIII)

1976. D (IX)

1977. C (X)

1978. A (XI)

1979. O (XII)

1980. M (XIII)

1981. G (XIV)

1982. B (XV)

1983. J (XVI)

1984. I (XVII)

REFERENCES

CHAPTER 34

I. P. M. Wax, "Sodium Bicarbonate," in *Goldfrank's Toxicologic Emergencies*, 9th ed., ed. L. S. Nelson et al. (New York: McGraw-Hill, 2011), 520–527.

II. M. A. Howland, "L-carnitine," in *Goldfrank's Toxicologic Emergencies*, 9th ed., ed. L. S. Nelson et al. (New York: McGraw-Hill, 2011), 711–713.

III. T. C. Bania, "Intravenous Fat Emulsions," in *Goldfrank's Toxicologic Emergencies*, 9th ed., ed. L. S. Nelson et al. (New York: McGraw-Hill, 2011), 976–981.

IV. M. A. Howland, "Glucagon," in *Goldfrank's Toxicologic Emergencies*, 9th ed., ed. L. S. Nelson et al. (New York: McGraw-Hill, 2011), 910–913.

V. Ibid., "Octeride," in *Goldfrank's Toxicologic Emergencies*, 9th ed., ed. L. S. Nelson el at. (New York: McGraw-Hill, 2011), 734–737.

VI. K. M. Sutin, "Dantrolene Sodium," in *Goldfrank's Toxicologic Emergencies*, 9th ed., ed. L. S. Nelson et al. (New York: McGraw-Hill, 2011), 1001–1002.

VII. R. S. Hoffman, "Prussian Blue," in *Goldfrank's Toxicologic Emergencies*, 9th ed., ed. L. S. Nelson et al. (New York: McGraw-Hill, 2011),1334—1338.

VIII. M. A. Howland, "Physostigmine Salicylate," in *Goldfrank's Toxicologic Emergencies*, 9th ed., ed. L. S. Nelson et al. (New York: McGraw-Hill, 2011), 759–762.

IX. Ibid., "Protamine," in *Goldfrank's Toxicologic Emergencies*, 9th ed., ed. L. S. Nelson et al. (New York: McGraw-Hill, 2011), 880–883.

X. Ibid., "Pyridoxine," in *Goldfrank's Toxicologic Emergencies*, 9th ed., ed. L. S. Nelson et al. (New York: McGraw-Hill, 2011), 845–848.

XI. Ibid., "Leucovorin(Folinic Acid) and Folic Acid," in *Goldfrank's Toxicologic Emergencies*, 9th ed., ed. L. S. Nelson et al. (New York: McGraw-Hill, 2011), 783–787.

XII. Ibid., "Flumazenil," in *Goldfrank's Toxicologic Emergencies*, 9th ed., ed. L. S. Nelson et al. (New York: McGraw-Hill, 2011), 1072–1077.

XIII. Ibid., "Fomepizole," in *Goldfrank's Toxicologic Emergencies*, 9th ed., ed. L. S. Nelson et al. (New York: McGraw-Hill, 2011), 1414–1419.

XIV. R. S. Hoffman, L. S. Nelson, and M. A. Howland, "Benzodiazepines," in *Goldfrank's Toxicologic Emergencies*, 9th ed., ed. L. S. Nelson et al. (New York: McGraw-Hill, 2011), 1109–1114.

XV. M. A. Howland, "Atropine," in *Goldfrank's Toxicologic Emergencies*, 9th ed., ed. L. S. Nelson et al. (New York: McGraw-Hill, 2011), 1473–1476.

XVI. Ibid., "Calcium," in *Goldfrank's Toxicologic Emergencies*, 9th ed., ed. L. S. Nelson et al. (New York: McGraw-Hill, 2011), 1381–1385.

XVII. J. G. Rella, "DPTA[Pentetic Acid or Pentate (Zinc or Calcium) Trisodium]," in *Goldfrank's Toxicologic Emergencies*, 9th ed., ed. L. S. Nelson et al. (New York: McGraw-Hill, 2011), 1779–1781.

35

TOXICOLOGIC DISASTERS

Matching Test

1985. sulfanilamide disaster 1937

1986. Love Canal, 1973-1975

1987. Bhopal, India, 1984

1988. Seveso, Italy, 1976

1989. Xiaoying, China, 2003

1990. Turkey, 1956

1991. Spain, 1981

1992. Minamata Bay, Japan, 1950s

1993. Japan, 1968

1994. Chicago, United States, 1982

1995. Chernobyl, Ukrane, 1986

1996. United States, 1989

1997. Europe, 1960s

1998. Pittsburgh, United States, 1988

1999. United States, 1930-1931

2000. San Jose, United States, 1982

A. hydrogen sulfide

B. hexachlorobenzene

C. PCBs

D. tylenol-cyanide

E. radiation sickness

F. L-tryptophan eosinophilia-myalgia syndrome

G. methyl isocyanate

H. thalidomide

I. China white epidemic

J. ethylene glycol

K. Ginger Jake paralysis

L. MPTP

M. kepone

N. dioxin

O. methylmercury

P. toxic oil syndrome

CHAPTER 35 ANSWERS (REFERENCES)

1985.   J (I)
1986.   M (I)
1987.   G (I)
1988.   N (I)
1989.   A (I)
1990.   B (I)
1991.   P (I)
1992.   O (I)
1993.   C (I)
1994.   D (I)
1995.   E (I)
1996.   F (I)
1997.   H (I)
1998.   I (I)
1999.   K (I)
2000.   L (I)

REFERENCES

CHAPTER 35

I. P. M. Wax, "Toxicologic Plagues and Disasters in History," in *Goldfrank's Toxicologic Emergencies*, 9th ed., ed. L. S. Nelson et al. (New York: McGraw-Hill, 2011), 18–30.

ABOUT THE AUTHOR

Dr. Richard J. Fruncillo spent most of his professional career as a clinical pharmacologist/human toxicologist conducting phase 1 clinical research studies for a major US pharmaceutical corporation. In addition to being a practicing internal medicine physician, he has an undergraduate degree in chemistry and a PhD in biochemical pharmacology. He is certified by the American Board of Internal Medicine, the American Board of Clinical Pharmacology, and the American Board of Toxicology. He has previously taught pharmacology/toxicology at the medical/graduate school level and is the author of many scientific publications in the areas of basic and clinical pharmacology/toxicology. Currently, he is a consultant to the medical and legal professions in the areas of pharmacology, toxicology, and drug development.